SEXUAL ECSTAS.

Also by Margot Anand

The Art of Sexual Ecstasy
The Art of Sexual Magic

SEXUAL ECSTASY

THE ART OF ORGASM

MARGOT ANAND

ILLUSTRATED BY ATMA PRITI

EXERCISES FROM *The Art of Sexual Magic*

JEREMY P. TARCHER/PUTNAM
A MEMBER OF
PENGUIN PUTNAM INC.
NEW YORK

Most Tarcher/Putnam books are available at special quantity
discounts for bulk purchase for sales promotions, premiums,
fund-raising, and educational needs. Special books or book
excerpts also can be created to fit specific needs.
For details, write Putnam Special Markets, 375 Hudson Street,
New York, NY 10014.

The exercises in this book have previously been published in
The Art of Sexual Magic copyright 1995 by Margo Anand, aka
M. E. Naslednikov.

Jeremy P. Tarcher/Putnam
a member of
Penguin Putnam Inc.
375 Hudson Street
New York, NY 10014
www.penguinputnam.com

Library of Congress Cataloging-in-Publication Data

Anand, Margot.
Sexual ecstasy : the art of orgasm / Margot Anand ; illustrated by Atma
Priti.
p. cm.
ISBN 1-58542-028-X
1. Sex instruction. 2. Female orgasm. 3. Sex—Religious aspects—
Tantrism. I. Title.
HQ64.A69   2000   00-023422
613.9'6—dc21
Printed in the United States of America

1 3 5 7 9 10 8 6 4 2

This book is printed on acid-free paper. ∞

Book design by Tanya Maiboroda
Illustrations by Atma Priti

A Word of Caution

The purpose of this book is to educate. It is not intended to give medical or psychological therapy. Whenever there is concern about physical or emotional illness, a qualified professional should be consulted.

All the sexual positions, rituals, and activities in this book are not for every body. Some of the positions were accomplished only after years of yogic practice.

Because of the litigation-happy times in which we live, here is the necessary legal disclaimer:

The author, illustrator, and publisher shall have neither liability nor responsibility to any person or entity with respect to any loss, damage, injury, or ailment caused or alleged to be caused directly or indirectly by the information or lack of information in this book.

So take responsibility for your own health. Please don't get stuck in a position you can't get out of.

CONTENTS

INTRODUCTION

What is this mysterious power in sexual love that thrills and electrifies us, that puts a "spring in our step" and makes us feel vibrant and alive? It is more than physical sensations shared between bodies, though this is essential for "good sex." It is the intensely pleasurable surging in us of a life force that is physical, creative, and even spiritual. The fact is that our bodies are designed to experience incredible pleasure that can take us to the roots of our creativity, and to the heights of spiritual awareness. And sex is how we get there.

The Multi-Orgasmic Response (MORE) training

presented in this book provides keys for you, and your lover, to unlock, through your most intimate encounters, an inner "pleasure chest" of untapped riches. It will help you develop those skills and qualities that can make you a great lover, and which make truly ecstatic lovemaking possible.

Yet, inner obstacles stand in the way. There is a taboo at the root of our being, a deep shame and guilt embedded in our psyches and our sex that rob us of our power, our freedom, and our ecstasy. A myth haunts us: Adam and Eve's exile from the Garden. Their "sin"—self-knowledge, even pleasure itself, we are told—implicitly becomes our own each time we climb into bed with our lover. Yet love is God in action; sex is love in motion; and we can, through acts of love, bring about God, and ecstasy, in our personal lives. Our sexual wounds can be healed. And in that healing, we reclaim the incredible generative/creative power that also lives at the root of who we are. Through self-knowledge, even through ecstatic sexual pleasure itself, we can return to the Garden. This is the purpose of the MORE sexual practices taught in this book.

So what elements make truly ecstatic lovemaking possible? Love, for one. But love alone isn't enough. Other qualities are essential: A relaxed body, attuned to feeling.

A heart opened in trust. A mind that is peaceful, present, and clear of negative thinking. A spiritual/sensual connection to yourself and your partner. Self-knowledge, even at the level of the physical body. The ability to direct your energy through breathing. And finally, precise technical skills in the art of loving, which can, and often must, be learned. Love, of course, can't be taught. But the MORE training will teach you how to practice and develop the rest.

Developing these skills will require committment and patience. To achieve maximum results, I suggest that you make a formal committment, to yourself and with your partner, and create a practice schedule. I recommend a minimum of two 30 to 90 minute "practice sessions" per week at fixed times—perhaps once on the weekend, and one evening in the middle of the week, though you can do more if you like. It helps to remember that this is the "practice" of receiving and giving erotic pleasure, and the skills you develop are those of all great lovers.

Also, this is a step-by-step training. It is important to fully and patiently engage each step, and to notice and address any "issues" it brings up, before moving on to the next. Be gentle. Don't push yourself, or your partner. Respect your concerns, fears, and apparent limits. Move gently through them at a pace that feels comfortable and right for you. It is also useful to keep a journal of any insights and experiences generated through this practice. Self-knowledge is precious, and a record of your progress may be invaluable later on.

Finally, creating a sacred space for your intimate practice with your beloved is essential. The room should be your temple, clean, uncluttered, and sensually arranged. Colors, textures, sounds, scents, and imagery, artistically combined, can create a potent environment that evokes and enhances moods of eros, harmony, sensuality, and love. Use beautiful rugs, sensual fabrics such as silk or velvet robes, sheets, and bedspreads. Wear sexy underwear and exotic kimonos. Surround yourself with powerful paintings, photographs, or sculptures. Enliven the atmosphere with plants, candles or soft lighting, sensual oils, incense, flowers, and beautiful music. Adequate space is important for stretching, moving, even dancing, in preparation for erotic play. If your bedroom is too small, perhaps temporarily transform a den or living room into your temple of love.

In this MORE training, you will be learning precise and powerful techniques of sexual massage. You will learn how to stimulate the orgasmic trigger points of both male and female genitals *(In this book I call the penis a "vajra" and the vagina a "yoni." I use these classical tantric terms to break the limiting mental associations we tend to have toward the more familiar terms. Their ritual meanings will be explained in the text.);* and how to maintain deep attention/relaxation during states of intense sexual and emotional arousal. These practices initiate deep physical and emotional contact between you and your partner, and so develop intimacy and trust. They also develop sexual prowess and the ability to experience extended, whole-body orgasm.

These methods have been widely tested. I have taught the MORE training to thousands of couples around the world for well over a decade—both heterosexual and same-sex couples—as well as single individuals. And these methods have delivered consistent and significant benefits to both men and women. One key benefit for women is the ability to become sexually aroused more quickly and fully, and to experience whole-body orgasm through sexual intercourse . . . an achievement that, according to statistics, eludes the majority of women, who must often "come by other means." A key benefit of this practice for men is an increased ability to control ejaculation in states of "high arousal," and even to experience extended, whole-body orgasm itself without ejaculation.

Yet in this practice, the term "high arousal" includes not only states of intense sexual/spiritual pleasure, but states of intense emotion of any kind. The MORE training confronts all deeply ingrained taboos against self-knowledge and pleasure. This practice may stir up primal feelings that have limited your ability to experience ecstatic states of deep intimacy and whole-body pleasure. These feelings may include fear, guilt, shame, sadness, or feelings of inadequacy or unworthiness—often related to past failed relationships or personal/cultural taboos against pleasure itself. The highest degree of pleasure, or ecstasy, requires the most explicit self-knowledge. And you will learn in this practice to be compassionately present to all of your feelings in peace, in the healing presence of your lover.

A truly great lover is also part healer, and part initiator. And the MORE practice is as much about healing as about ecstasy, and as much about spirit as about sex. It allows the relaxation of unconscious emotional/sexual anxiety we may have carried for years; and relaxation of a corresponding physical armoring around the genitals, which many people carry throughout their lives. Both "tensions" inhibit our ability to experience true whole-body pleasure and ecstatic sexual intimacy. And such ecstasy itself can heal deep sexual and emotional wounds.

In this training you will also learn the Three Keys to orgasmic power, and the Five Virtues of ecstatic lovers. The Three Keys are: 1) Breathing with attention. 2) Movement with feeling. 3) Voice with expression. People who feel inhibited or non-orgasmic during lovemaking are usually trapped in their minds and cut off from sensual and emotional feeling. These conditions are reenforced by shallow breathing. Proper breathing relaxes and energizes the body, clarifies and focuses the mind, and opens us up to new depths of sensual/emotional feeling, which can then be expressed and enhanced through vocal expression. When we are so "attuned," our speech becomes eros, part of the play of our lovemaking. We can guide our lover verbally in their pleasuring of us, and also "sing" the notes of our pleasure in ecstatic communion with our lover.

The Five Virtues of ecstatic lovers developed through the Multi-Orgasmic Response training benefit every area of life. They are:

Patience: Lovemaking, like any art or skill, involves learning. Patience is therefore essential. Sex, like love, cannot be hurried. Yet the restless mind tends to want everything now, and to rush through each moment at the "speed of thought" toward an imagined goal. Impatience disturbs the body's sensual rhythms, the ebb and flow in the rising cycles of lovemaking. It disrupts awareness, separating us from ourselves and our lover. This leads to disappointment, frustration, and even anger. Patience allows us to meet each moment without struggle or reaction, and to avoid this negative or anti-ecstatic cycle. Patience is also the virtue that opens the door to Trust, Presence, and Compassion.

Trust: Without Trust, intimacy is not possible, and pleasure cannot rise to the level of ecstasy. Trust here includes trust in yourself. Trust in the knowledge that you are lovable and deserve pleasure. Trust in your lover's essential goodness, and their good intentions with you. Trust in the healing, transforming power of sex. Trust in life itself, as your guide and teacher in each moment of experience. Trust lets us open in surrender, be vulnerable and receptive, rather than armored and defensive in the most intimate acts of love. Trust allows us to enter the cycles of giving and receiving, fully and wholeheartedly.

Presence: Presence is the quality of being authentic, fully present in attention, emotion, body, and breath. Presence allows us to fully experience the physical touch, and emotional presence of our lover. Without Presence, our mind roams, emotional contact with our partner is broken, awareness of our own body and its sensations is lost, and the act of love becomes mechanical. Presence unlocks an essential vitality and receptivity that allow sex to merge with spirit. And this communion of sex and spirit is the essence of ecstatic lovemaking.

Compassion: Compassion is the basis of unconditional love. Compassion never demands perfection of self or others, but blesses wholeheartedly regardless of apparent shortcomings or flaws. (There is no room for judgment in the Garden.) When we have Compassion for ourselves as we are, especially in the often "wounded" area of sexuality, we can grant the same regard to our lover. Compassion heals those gaps when you or your lover do not know what to do, or feel awkward, embarrassed, uncertain, or are unable to receive or give pleasure. In such moments, Compassion melts away tensions, restores harmony, and opens the door to the next level of intimacy and pleasure.

Clarity: Clarity awakens when we are Patient, Trusting, Present, and Compassionately related to ourselves and our lover. Clarity allows us to notice and express our needs explicitly, without complication or inhibition—to be simple and direct, in our words, our sounds, and our bodily expressions. In Clarity, we become eloquent at the level of wordless communication. In Clarity, we know our own needs, and can teach our lover how to satisfy them. This is how we help them to become great lovers.

These Three Keys and Five Virtues also empower us in our daily life. For self-mastery in the bedroom translates into mastery in living. When we can remain calm, present, trusting, relaxed, compassionate, and clear in the most vulnerable and highly charged arena of sexual intimacy, we can also maintain these qualities amidst the crises and stresses of daily life.

This practice will also release in you tremendous energy formerly bound up in unconscious internal conflicts. This energy is not just sexual, but creative in the highest sense. Sexuality is the creative life force itself, and its release initiates us into new levels of creativity, freedom, and personal power. Not to mention new levels of sexual mastery. These skills will allow you to choose with expanded awareness, and offer with greater skill, that true joy and pleasure that lead both you and your beloved to ecstasy.

Skillful lovers become divine instruments in a symphony of delight. Their communion *is* ecstasy, the highest state of self-knowing, and self-forgetting. Their loving heals all wounds, washes away the stresses of living, and eases the burden of being an apparently limited personality in a world of apparent limits, threats, and taboos.

And as they reenter the Garden through their ecstasy, Spirit is there to welcome them; and perhaps to ask, "What took you so long?"

MORE
The Multi-Orgasmic Response for Women

Every woman knows that she holds inside herself a tremendous capacity for love. This love can take many forms—from the nurturing mother to the devoted partner in a committed relationship to the wild and ecstatic lover. For a woman to open herself to this love, to expand into it, to be fulfilled by it, is perhaps the greatest magic that she can accomplish.

The key to opening the door of love is expanded sexual orgasm. This is the root of the woman's tree of love, her earthly base, her dark, fertile, hidden source of vital energy out of which her tree can grow to great heights, blossoming in spectacular abundance with the wonderful, fragrant flowers of love.

At the risk of making the rest of this book seem almost redundant, I have to say that a truly orgasmic woman needs no other tools for magic. Her radiance, her bubbling energy, her sexual vitality, her overflowing heart, make her so magnetically attractive that she naturally and effortlessly draws to herself everything that she needs.

But how many women can claim to know this magical state, which is both our potential and our birthright? Even today, in a relatively liberal culture that has become aware of the repression of women and is beginning to undo the damage inflicted by centuries of male domination, the art of attaining full satisfying orgasmic states remains frustratingly elusive for the vast majority of women.

In this book, women learn the secrets of how to experience intense, prolonged, and ecstatic orgasms, while their male partners learn the delicate art of giving this ultimate pleasure to their beloved. And, should this task seem too one-sided, men can take comfort in the knowledge that in the following chapter they will learn the secrets of expanding male orgasm. For just as most women have been denied their potential for orgasmic pleasure, so the majority of men have settled for something less than true sexual fulfillment, contenting themselves with a local,

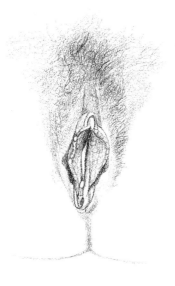

Yoni "au naturel"

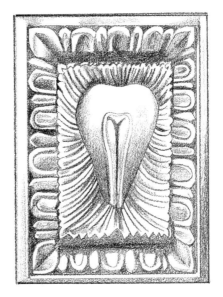

Icon of the yoni emanating rays of energy. From a South Indian wood carving of the nineteenth century.

genital, ejaculatory release instead of bathing in the exquisite sensations of total orgasm.

You are now ready to generate the maximum amount of orgasmic power as an alchemical fuel for your transformation, using the full spectrum of your orgasmic sensations to change your vision and give it tremendous potency.

Without this incredibly powerful energy, the ceremony and ritual of love look rather like a beautiful auto-

Venus yields to caresses, not to compulsion.

—PUBLILIUS
Moral Sayings

mobile that has no engine. Its appearance is magnificent, your neighbors can admire it, but it cannot go anywhere. Sexual orgasm provides the engine, the horsepower, the pulsing, dynamic force that transforms love into magic.

In this chapter you will be focusing on the fundamentals of expanding orgasm. You will also discover that, in the process of increasing your orgasmic potential, a profound healing will take place in your capacity to relate intimately with your beloved. As you will see, when two love partners move through the delicate stages that lead to expanded orgasm, and through the equally important steps of helping each other attain this experience, they learn every element needed for an intense and fulfilling relationship, including deep communication, courage, honesty, sensitivity, and trust.

Healing the Past

Today, women's psyches are still influenced by centuries of patriarchal repression. This means that, until recently, we were programmed by a male-dominated society to believe that our main purpose in life was to service the needs and pleasures of the man, particularly in regard to sex. His pleasure was paramount, both in terms of his immediate sexual gratification and his goal of creating male heirs to inherit his name, his property, and his social status. If women got any sexual pleasure at all, it was in the form of crumbs that fell from the man's plate while he was eating.

During this time, most women had no idea that such a thing as female orgasm existed and, if they did, they were usually intelligent enough to keep quiet about it. The last thing men wanted to know was that their "inferior" partners were capable of experiencing more sexual pleasure than they permitted themselves.

All this has been well documented, and there is no need to cover this sad and painful story again. However, in terms of fulfilling orgasmic potential, it is important for women to understand that they still carry the legacy of this conditioning, especially in the delicate area of sexual satisfaction.

This legacy has its origins in our religious roots, in the historical shift that occurred when patriarchal religions like Judaism, Christianity and Islam succeeded in wiping out all forms of worship devoted to a female or mother goddess. As part of this victory, female sexuality was condemned. It had to be, because the very essence of the religion of the mother goddess was fertility and the renewal of life through sexual union. Through the goddess, sexuality had a natural, sacred role to play in religion and therefore in society.

Eros is the force that draws a child to lie in its mother's lap, that evokes magical passion between lovers of all ages, the force that in its higher manifestation attracts souls to love. Eros is the power of the shakti. Eros is the child of Aphrodite.

—ANDREW HARVEY

To a significant extent, the annihilation of the mother goddess depended on the ability of the patriarchal priesthood to condemn sex and make people feel guilty about their natural sexual feelings. And, in a cunning strategy that has to be admired for its enduring impact, the priests and prophets succeeded in creating a powerful myth that made women responsible for our sexual shame, thus further eradicating the influence of the mother goddess in religious practice.

Through propagating the myth of Adam and Eve, the priests showed how the first woman tempted the first man to commit the original sin. It was Eve who encouraged Adam to disobey Jehovah and eat from the Tree of Knowledge.

And what was the first dawning of their knowledge? Not a sudden understanding of the laws of nature, such as how to create fire or shape a wheel. Not the discovery of music, poetry, dance, or painting. No, the first "knowledge" that came to Adam and Eve was the discovery that they were naked. In other words, that they were sexual beings. They had genitals, sexual organs, a vagina or a penis, and these they shamefully covered with fig leaves.

This legacy of shame, of condemnation, lives on in the subconscious minds of all women. Even today, when asserting their equality with men, there is a strong tendency for women to prove their worth by imitating men and competing with them for success in a patriarchal society, rather than through acknowledging and reembracing their truly female qualities.

Sexually, this tendency manifests itself as an effort to meet the man in a contest of sexual athletics, with both partners focusing on performance and achievement, striving for excitement and release. The woman may succeed in having an orgasm, but through this approach it usually remains superficial. It does not go deep. It does not flood her very being with the ecstasy of which she is capable.

Beneath a surface layer of liberated attitudes, women still carry a deep wound around their sexuality. All kinds of deep-seated beliefs and fears inhibit the natural flow of their orgasmic energy. Beliefs such as "I can't ask for what I want because I don't deserve it," or "I shouldn't be feeling this pleasure," or "It's the man's role to give me pleasure, and I must settle for what he gives me," and fears such as "If I really let go into my orgasmic energy, he'll think I'm too much."

In my work with women during the past fifteen years I have discovered that this is their constantly recurring dark secret: the belief that they are not worthy of receiving pleasure and, since they are not important, they can gain value only by serving and pleasing the man. It is time to remedy this imbalanced state of affairs. It is time for women to experience the true liberation as female sexual beings.

THE HEALING ALCHEMY OF ORGASM

The damage caused to human society by the condemnation of sex is incalculable. Instead of accepting sexual union of women and men as a natural, healthy, and blissful act, we have turned sex into a furtive, guilt-ridden affair. Instead of celebrating sex as the creative, fertile life force that it really is, we have tried to hide it behind locked doors and even to pretend that it does not exist.

The effects of this misguided attitude stretch far beyond lovemaking and even beyond the flood tide of pornography, prostitution, rape, sexual abuse, and sexual harassment that our society is currently experiencing. It influences our entire worldview.

For example, these days, a tremendous amount of well-intentioned effort is being made to heal the global environment, to stop the destruction of our planetary biosphere, to bring peace to warring ethnic, national, and religious factions.

Yet, how can any of this happen when the very source of human love is poisoned? How can love for the planet and love for each other flourish and prosper when the basic teaching of organized religion is that the sexual life force itself is evil, that our flesh is corrupted, that a vast and unbridgeable gap exists between the world of spirit and the world of earthly pleasure?

Intellectually, we may feel that we have discarded damaging myths such as Eve's original sin, but we need only look at the wounded state of human sexual behavior to realize that this ancient propaganda still lives in the subconscious part of our minds. The old paradigm has not yet been replaced. We have not yet stepped out of the prison of patriarchal history.

Fortunately, there are effective and simple ways to free ourselves from this primitive programming. For woman, the road to true sexual liberation consists of walking the sacred path that begins with the first stirrings of sexual pleasure in her genitals and ends in a prolonged and thoroughly fulfilling orgasm. With this creative act of cherishing her body, encouraging her own ecstasy, the woman can reconnect with the goddess within, not as some mythical deity but as the living principle of female wholeness.

The reemergence of the sacred feminine principle goes hand in hand with the rebirth of the feminine pleasure principle, and with the balancing of male and female prerogatives to the experience of sexual pleasure.

The sexual ecstasy of a woman has a very high value. It is a magical, healing force. When she has been well loved, sexually fulfilled, she herself becomes a goddess with magical powers—radiating love, devotion, caring, gratitude, happiness. She has the capacity to restore the life force of sex to its rightful place in the temple of human understanding, opening the way for planetary healing and transformation.

An important part of this healing is the recognition that the male and female principles are not opposites, locked in an endless struggle for domination, but complementaries whose destiny is to unite in a Tantric dance of energy, flooding both partners with orgasmic joy.

Healing also comes in the form of a deep understanding between man and woman. In the following exercises, both partners learn new forms of communication. The woman, especially, learns to ask for what she wants, teaching her partner how to give her pleasure. She will be defining her sensations, recognizing any resistance that may surface as she rises to heightened states of orgasmic pleasure, learning the art of surrender and letting go into ecstasy.

The man learns how to caress and stimulate his love partner's sexual organ, taking her to new peaks of excitement. In doing so, he will experience the immense satisfaction that comes from voluntarily and gladly serving the other, gaining a deep appreciation of the interdependence that exists between a man and a woman when they move into lovemaking as true equals.

Only out of such equality can both partners experience their complementary roles as cocreators of ecstasy.

Anatomy of Female Orgasm: The Clitoris and the G-Spot

Before introducing the alchemy designed to enhance a woman's experience of orgasm, I would like to describe the physical anatomy of the female sexual organ. As I explained in *The Art of Sexual Ecstasy,* a sound working knowledge of the genitals is essential for those who wish to expand their orgasmic potential.

You will be exploring two orgasmic trigger points in the female sexual organ: the clitoris, which is the source of external or clitoral orgasm, and the so-called G-Spot, which is the source of a deeper, vaginal orgasm. You will be learning how to stimulate these points, first separately, then together in a blended orgasm that can fill the whole pelvic area and even your entire body.

Thinking always of the Goddess, one is transformed into an image of the Goddess.
　　　　—HINDU TANTRA

Female readers are invited to treat the following description as an exercise by sitting down in front of a mirror and exploring the vagina as I describe it. Men can study the vagina of their partners, who may want to recline comfortably on cushions and open their legs, inviting the man to explore this normally invisible area of female sexuality.

The vagina is surrounded and protected by soft folds of skin called the labia. When these are spread back, you can see the mouth of the vagina, which leads into the vaginal canal (see illustration, page 13). Above the mouth of the vagina, at the point where the labia meet, or sometimes a little higher, is the clitoris.

The clitoris looks like a small round pearl or button. It is covered by a hood of skin which, when pulled back, reveals the tip of this delicate mechanism. There is a shaft, just below the tip, that divides into leglike parts that run on either side of the vaginal canal. Although you can see only the tip, you can feel the shaft just beneath the surface of the skin.

According to well-established research, a large majority of women who experience orgasm do so through manual stimulation of the clitoris, either by themselves or by a partner. Only a small minority of women experience clitoral orgasm during penetration by the penis, and even

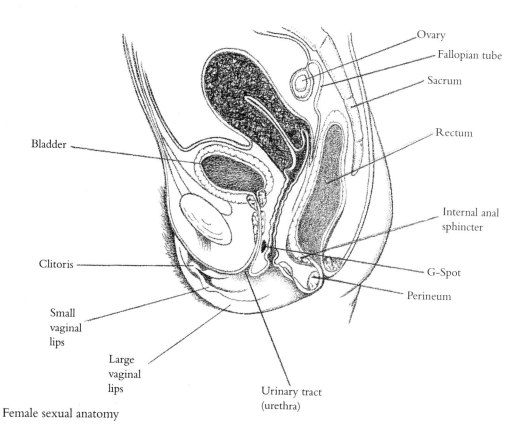

Female sexual anatomy

fewer experience a deeper orgasm inside the vagina. That is why it is so important to know how to stimulate the clitoris before sexual penetration.

As you can easily discover by gently touching its tip, the clitoris is quite mobile. It can and does move around during lovemaking, sliding in and out of the vaginal opening. When a woman becomes sexually aroused the clitoris enlarges to approximately double its size, but when she gets really excited and approaches sexual climax the clitoris tends to retract until hidden once more under the clitoral hood. If the woman becomes less excited, but still aroused, the clitoris will reappear.

The anatomy of a woman's clitoris can vary greatly. In her book *Sex for One,* Betty Dodson relates that when a group of women gathered to view and compare their sexual organs they discovered that "when the hood was pulled back and each clitoris appeared, the variations were astounding, ranging from tiny little seed pearls, to rather large and protruding jewels."

Members of Dodson's group found no relationship between the size of the clitoris and the degree of pleasure of which it was capable. It was not a question of the bigger the clitoris, the better the orgasm. All sizes seemed to perform well, when correctly pleasured.

The most remarkable thing about the clitoris, as many women know, is its incredible sensitivity. As you will discover in the first exercise of this chapter, the more this pleasure trigger is stimulated the more responsive and sensitive it becomes.

The second orgasmic trigger point in a woman's

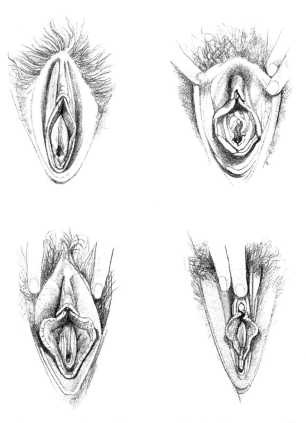

Different types of Yonis showing how varied female sexual anatomy can be, after Betty Dodson's drawings from *Sex for One*

sexual organ is the G-Spot, named after Ernst von Gra-fenberg, the German physician who discovered it. The G-Spot lies inside the vagina, behind the pubic bone, on the roof of the vaginal canal.

The best way to locate the G-Spot is to rest a finger on the tip of the clitoris, then trace the finger slowly down, entering the mouth of the vagina at the top of the opening, then moving the finger inside for a distance of about one and a half to two inches, staying on the roof of the vaginal canal. The telltale mark of the G-Spot is that the tissue here feels ribbed or rigid, like a small button with tiny bumps on it, whereas the rest of the vaginal walls are smooth. The best time to feel the G-Spot is soon after a woman has experienced orgasm, when it becomes somewhat enlarged and more sensitive.

There are several theories about why the G-Spot is sensitive, the most interesting being that the nerves that provide pleasure at the clitoris pass through this area on their way to the spine. There is also a nerve connection between the G-Spot and the bladder, resulting in an illusory impression that you need to urinate when this area is stimulated.

The G-Spot is surrounded by spongy tissue known as the "glands of Bartholin" which, when stimulated, may release prostatic-type fluids in the form of female ejaculation.

Attaining sexual arousal and orgasm through massaging the G-Spot is a delicate art which I will describe in the second exercise of this chapter. Having mastered the art of stimulating both the clitoris and the G-Spot you will be ready to explore a blended, expanded orgasm created by pleasuring both spots simultaneously.

In this way, the practice of expanded orgasm is given in three steps:

1. Clitoral stimulation and clitoral orgasm

2. G-Spot stimulation and vaginal orgasm

3. Simultaneous stimulation of clitoris and G-Spot leading to an expanded or blended orgasm

Once you have acquired the necessary skills, you can do all three steps in a single session.

OVERCOMING INITIAL EMBARRASSMENT

It can be quite scary for a woman to open her legs and allow a man to examine her Yoni, her vagina. There is something about the delicate act of exposing the genitals to detailed inspection that triggers feelings of insecurity vulnerability, and embarrassment.

In normal lovemaking, the woman is filled with reassuring sensations as she is taken by the man and held in close body contact while he caresses her Yoni and penetrates with his Vajra. But in this exercise both the man and the woman are adopting an approach that is almost scien-

Look upon a woman as a Goddess, whose special energy she is, and honor her in that state of Goddess.

—UTARA TANTRA

17

tific. It is rather like taking a magnifying glass and holding it in front of the genitals, revealing not only the physical anatomy but also any attitudes you may carry about your sexual organ and your right to sexual pleasure—whether you deserve it, whether you can allow it and surrender to it.

In spite of these doubts, you are going to give yourself permission to lie back and receive, allowing a man to pleasure you for as long as it takes to feel totally orgasmic. You deserve this moment. You have waited patiently for it long enough.

And the beauty of it is that, although you are vulnerable and receptive during this exercise, you, the woman, are in charge. You are the one who is going to discover how and where you like to be touched, exploring and bringing awareness to every millimeter of your sexual organ, teaching your beloved exactly how to caress each pleasure point.

Knowing that you are in charge will give you courage to move through any resistances that you encounter during clitoral stimulation, knowing that you can at any time stop or change the nature of the caresses that are being given to you.

One more thing: Many women experience that massaging the clitoris and the vagina heals and sensitizes scar tissue in the area, such as may be caused by a difficult childbirth. However, if you have an ongoing history of vaginal infection or other medical problems relating to your sexual organ, you should not do this massage unless you receive permission from your doctor.

EXERCISE: PLEASURING THE CLITORIS

Purpose and Benefits

As the receiver in this exercise, you, the woman, are about to experience one of the most challenging and ecstatic pleasuring sessions of your life. For centuries the clitoris has been a hidden part of our sexual anatomy, often disregarded as an unimportant, incomplete appendage. It has been our guilty secret, a place that only we know how to pleasure fully.

The majority of women do not realize that it is possible to teach a man how to pleasure this secret part skillfully and masterfully.

This exercise gives you full permission to enjoy and celebrate the sexual pleasure that arises from your clitoris, thereby healing any negative beliefs that you may have regarding your sexual organs.

As a woman, and as a magician, you are about to enter a new era that will enhance your self-esteem and embrace the alchemy of your orgasmic power. In this session, let the goddess of love blossom within you. You are worth it!

Know that the key for moving from good sex to great sex is to allow yourself to fully receive this gift while you encourage your man to give you exactly what you like. This, in turn, will validate his skills as a great lover.

This exercise will:

- Provide detailed knowledge of the female sexual organs.

- Bring new awareness to the areas where sexual pleasure is available and to ways of caressing these areas.

- Open the way for ecstatic states of sexual orgasm.

- Reveal and dissolve any psychological or emotional blocks that may inhibit the flow of orgasmic energy.

- Enhance communication between love partners, deepening their sense of intimacy.

- Teach you, the woman, how to take responsibility for your sexual well-being.

- Help you, the woman, to learn the art of trust.

- Teach you, the man, how to bring a woman to orgasmic ecstasy.

❧ Help you, the man, to feel validated as giver, supporter, and expert lover.

Preparations and Practice

❧ In this exercise you will be addressing each other by your magical names. Here, I will continue to use the names Shakti and Shiva, the deities of Tantric union.

❧ It can be fun and helpful to create an atmosphere of sexual anticipation before the exercise, as if preparing for a special date. Earlier in the day, Shiva can call Shakti on the phone and say whatever words may turn her on, like "I want you, I want your pleasure trickling down my fingers, I want your wetness, I want you to be totally open to me . . ."

❧ Shiva, you may want to buy Shakti some sexy underwear, to be worn at the appointed hour of the exercise. Or perhaps you may decide to take her out to a restaurant and flirt under the table, reaching with your hands to forbidden places. Find ways to generate an aura of sexual, erotic excitement between you and your partner. Be creative.

❧ Shiva, you are also the one who creates the Magic Circle, taking time to make the space beautiful, adorning it with things that Shakti loves. Bring colorful cushions, a nice sheet for her to lie on, some flowers, incense, and candles, put on soft, nonintrusive music in the background. You can also bring objects that will give your woman reassurance, such as a favorite teddy bear or certain tarot cards and, of course, her Magic Symbol. You can enhance your woman's sense of self-esteem and her love for you, when she sees how much care you have taken to create a safe and sacred environment to support her pleasure.

- Shakti, while Shiva is preparing the Magic Circle, take a relaxed shower or bath, caress your body with oil, put on a touch of perfume, give yourself the feeling that you deserve luxury and care, as if you are the most important person in the world. Wear something soft and silky, like a kimono-style gown that opens in front.

- Shiva and Shakti: proceed at your own pace through the exercise, mastering each stage in turn.

- It is a good idea to have a jug of water or fruit juice handy, as this can be thirsty work.

- The room needs to be warm enough to work without much clothing.

- There needs to be plenty of lubricant available. For massaging the clitoris, an oil-based lubricant like

Vaseline will be best because you may be stimulating
this area for quite a long time and water-based lubricants tend to dry up too quickly.

❦ Shiva, check that your fingernails are trimmed and
smooth.

❦ Shakti, make sure that your bladder is empty.

❦ Allow sixty to ninety minutes for this exercise and be
sure that you will not be interrupted.

STAGE 1: SENSUAL FOREPLAY

Shiva, when the room is prepared, bring Shakti into the
Magic Circle. Be gracious, playful, reassuring. This is a
good time to dance together for a few minutes, shaking
off any nervousness or tension.

Greet each other with a Heart Salutation.

Have a long Melting Hug, breathing deeply, in synchronicity together.

Shiva, gently remove Shakti's gown and invite her to
lie on the cushions. Or, if she wishes, let her keep the
gown on, parting it to reveal her thighs and pelvis.

Sit cross-legged on her left side, close to her body,
and take a few minutes to create a position that will be
comfortable for both of you. In my experience, the best
position for the exercise is as follows:

Oh, recluse, if you aspire to paradise, go fast to that place where dwells the woman of lust.

—KUTTNI MAHA TYAN TANTRA

Shakti, open your legs, resting, your left leg on a pillow that is placed on Shiva's left knee.

Shiva, rest your left elbow and forearm on the same pillow.

Shakti, rest your right knee on another pillow so that your legs are spread comfortably apart and your knees slightly bent.

Shiva, place a pillow on your right thigh, which will support your right forearm.

Shiva, ask Shakti, "Are you comfortable?" If not, experiment with other positions, adjusting the cushions, until both of you are comfortable.

Be sure that your lubricant is nearby, so that you can reach it easily later in the exercise.

Shiva and Shakti, close your eyes for a few moments and breathe deeply into your abdomens. Take time to become centered and focused on what is about to happen.

Shiva, tune into your partner. Rest your left hand gently on Shakti's Yoni and your right hand on her heart chakra in the middle of her chest. Gaze softly into her eyes and begin to breathe in harmony. Feel the love in your heart for this beloved friend who is making herself vulnerable to you.

Shiva, when you feel ready, begin to stroke and caress Shakti's whole body very lightly, either with your fingertips or with feathers. As you do so, encourage her to breathe deeply through her mouth while staying relaxed and receptive. Talk to her gently, reassuringly, whispering "Just relax, beloved, and receive this gift that I am bringing to you. There is nothing to do, no goal to reach . . . All is for your pleasure."

With light fingers, caress every part of Shakti's body. Touch her lips, her neck, her nipples, belly, pubic mound, tugging gently at her pubic hair, caress her thighs, her feet, making sure that you touch every part of her body, bringing love and reassurance to each area. There is no hurry.

Shakti, this is your opportunity to relax more deeply into a mood of receptivity, giving yourself permission to enjoy what is being showered on you, letting go of the feeling that you have to do anything or please anyone.

STAGE 2: TIMING YOUR APPROACH

Shiva, watch Shakti's body language, which will indicate when she is ready for you to begin massaging her sexual organ directly. Through your gentle caresses, she is becoming sexually awakened. Her thighs are likely to open even farther, exposing her Yoni, while her pelvis may begin to push up slightly, raising her hips off the sheet as she invites you to explore her genitals.

If you are not sure, ask Shakti, "Is this a good time, beloved?" She may nod, or give a little sigh of agreement, or perhaps say, "No, please, spend a little more time caressing around my neck and shoulders, that feels so good."

Shiva, remember that you are in a response mode, listening to Shakti's guidance, learning how to caress her in ways that bring the maximum amount of pleasure.

Shakti, you are receiving pleasure, guiding your partner as to how to touch you. Don't be afraid to say exactly what you want. This is the time to give yourself everything.

STAGE 3: TEASING THE CLITORIS

Shiva, cover the fingers of your right hand with plenty of lubricant. Begin to stroke Shakti's genitals lightly, caressing the surface of her Yoni, touching the upper ridges of the lips, very delicately, like a feather. Gently tug on the pubic hair. Place your hand so that it covers the whole Yoni and gently vibrate the hand.

Take the lips of the Yoni and spread them apart like the wings of a butterfly so that the Yoni is completely open, then pass your lubricated fingers around the inside of the lips, near the entrance of the vagina itself, and all around the clitoris, then softly blow warm air from your mouth on the open lips.

Close the lips of the Yoni, pressing them gently together and massaging the outside of the lips, from the bottom up toward the clitoris. Continue to massage inside the lips of the Yoni, lightly sliding up toward the pubic mound, then down toward the anus, using lots of lubricant.

Shiva, tease Shakti's cleo, her clitoris, with an occasional touch, a tickle or caress, giving her a suggestion of more, then move to some other area of the Yoni, as if to say "I promise you pleasure. With this touch, light as the wings of a bird in flight, I honor your tenderness, your sensitivity. With this touch I show you that I can be sensitive and caring, in tune with you, listening, calling forth your pleasure."

Using a lot of lubricant is very pleasurable for Shakti. When your fingers are dry, they tend to pull and drag the surface of her Yoni in an uncomfortable way.

STAGE 4: STIMULATING THE CLITORIS
Shiva, now you can begin to rub Shakti's cleo lightly, allowing it to remain covered by the folds of its hood. Begin softly, caressingly, then start to explore the following massage strokes that can bring so much sexual pleasure to a woman.

The Two-Finger Basic Stroke   Begin with the two-finger basic stroke. Your thumb and index finger rest at the point where the clitoris goes inside the body and is no longer visible, that is to say, just below the tip, where the shaft disappears beneath the skin.

In this position, you are holding the shaft between your thumb and index finger and can roll it lightly between them. Experiment until you find this point and then slowly begin to massage evenly, rubbing up and down on either side of the shaft, finding a comfortable rhythm. For many women, the best timing is one stroke per second.

This movement has been called the "bread and butter stroke" because it is the easiest and simplest way of giving pleasure to a woman through her cleo.

Ask Shakti, "How does this feel?" Encourage her to give feedback, to tell you what kind of touch brings her the most pleasure.

The Double Stroke   After a while, try another stroke.

Rub up and down one side of the shaft with your thumb, while your index finger makes light circular motions on the other side.

The Rooted Stroke   Rest your thumb motionless on one side of the clitoral shaft and, using your index finger,

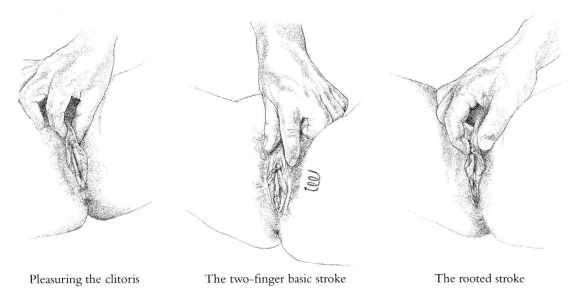

Pleasuring the clitoris   The two-finger basic stroke   The rooted stroke

caress the other side with small circular motions, moving from the root to the tip.

The Top Rub   Hold the shaft of the cleo with your thumb and middle finger, and use your index finger to massage the tip of the cleo very lightly, still with the hood covering the tip.

The Three-Finger Tickle Stroke   Use your thumb and middle finger to hold the root of the cleo, leaving the index finger free to massage the tip of the cleo.

Directly Stimulating the Cleo   When Shakti is strongly aroused, pull back the hood of the cleo with your thumb and middle finger and directly stimulate the tip of the clitoris with your index finger, rubbing lightly and consistently.

Ask Shakti, "How does this feel? Do you want it stronger or lighter?" Remember, you can do this only when Shakti has become aroused and her cleo is engorged, otherwise direct contact on the tip is likely to be too strong to be really pleasurable.

When Shakti is aroused, the shaft and tip of the cleo become stiff and swollen, like a little mound that sticks out of the surrounding flesh. Using the same basic grip, you can make vertical strokes up and down the sides of this mound, almost as if you were stimulating an erect penis. Or you can pulse, squeezing rapidly, or use circular motions.

Using two or three fingers, you can achieve a surprising variety of movements.

Making an Inventory   Take time to explore all the variations available, giving each other continuous feedback.

Shakti, it is tempting to get lost in the pleasure you are receiving. You may find it difficult to speak, or lack

Shiva's finger moves around
the vaginal labia, making
tiny circular motions from
the cleo (twelve o'clock)
down toward the perineum
(six o'clock).

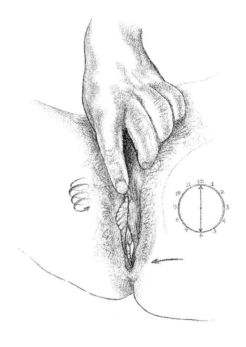

words to communicate with Shiva. But it is important for
you to stay aware of each sensation, expressing how you
feel, what you like, what you want to change. Communication is very important here.

This is a work of great art. You are teaching Shiva
the delicate skills of generating orgasmic arousal on a
tremendously sensitive but small part of your body.

Give feedback on each stroke or caress you receive.

If this is difficult, ask Shiva to repeat one stroke for about a minute, staying on the same point with the same rhythm while you find words to describe how this feels. When you are ready, move to another stroke, proceeding systematically as if learning a type of massage.

Shakti, you are looking for a point that can be very tiny, where the most pleasurable sensations arise. It can be a little circular motion on the right side of the clitoris shaft, or a thumb and index finger moving up and down the shaft on both sides.

Take time to make an inventory of strokes and rhythms that are pleasurable.

The Pleasure Clock   Going "around the clock" while caressing the Yoni can be a very helpful image in locating areas that are especially pleasurable on or near the cleo.

Shiva, with your mind's eye, imagine that a clock dial surrounds Shakti's cleo, so that the highest point, nearest her pubic mound, is the twelve o'clock position and the lowest point, nearest her vaginal opening, is the six o'clock position.

Move around the clock with your fingers, exploring each point. Make tiny circular motions with your index finger. When Shakti moans with pleasure, let her know "This is at three o'clock," or "This is at nine o'clock."

STAGE 5: BUILDING AROUSAL IN STEPS

Shiva, when you feel that you have mastered the various strokes for massaging Shakti's cleo, choose one and stay with this stroke for several minutes. Now you can explore your ability to raise Shakti's level of sexual excitement steadily.

Bring Shakti toward a peak of excitement with a slow, steady rhythm of about one stroke per second. Then, when she is on the edge of orgasm, slow down so that she has time to relax and absorb this energy.

Shakti, you can help Shiva know when to slow down by saying "I'm very close now."

Shiva, when Shakti is ready, increase stimulation again to help her move to an even higher level of pleasure, then slow down again. This is like helping Shakti to walk up a series of orgasmic steps, each one more pleasurable than the last.

The Pleasure Rating System

Shakti, one way to let Shiva know your level of arousal is to communicate via a zero-to-ten pleasure rating system.

For example, if you say "three," this tells Shiva that you are mildly aroused. If you say "six," this lets him know that you are getting really turned on, and a "nine" warns him that you are very close to orgasm. A "ten" means that you have gone over the orgasmic edge.

Shiva, watch carefully so that you can learn how to "read" Shakti's level of arousal. As she gets more and more excited, watch for the following signs:

1. Nipples becoming stiffer and darker

2. Pushing down and out with her pelvis

3. Arching her back

4. Flexing her toes and fingers

5. Vaginal opening becomes dark and engorged with blood

6. Vaginal canal becomes more visible

7. Clitoris becomes more stiff and exposed

Spreading Orgasmic Energy

Shiva, when Shakti's sexual excitement gets very strong, spread the sexual energy by moving your fingers down the outer lips of the vagina, stroking to the base near the anus, caressing up and down in this manner.

Shakti, you can also help to spread your orgasmic energy. Breathe deeply, letting each exhalation go down all the way to your Yoni. Caress your belly, your breasts, your shoulders. You will find that there is a sexual connection between your nipples and your cleo, and you may like to caress and squeeze them.

The woman you love, you must not possess.

—AZUL

Stay relaxed and receptive. When you feel really aroused you may be tempted to strive for orgasmic release, but see if you can relax into this energy that is awakening in you, letting it spread through your pelvis, rather than tensing up and striving for the explosive orgasm of release.

If you feel your sensations are becoming too intense, ask Shiva to slow the rhythm of his massage, change the stroke, or move his fingers to some other part of your Yoni. If it feels just right, say "Yes, yes!" or make pleasurable sounds. Vocalizing helps to increase your arousal level and conveys a message of encouragement to your partner.

STAGE 6: ORGASM OF THE CLITORIS
Shakti, you will know that you are approaching orgasm when you feel a tingling, buzz, or current of excitement

coming from deep inside, at the root of your clitoris, rising steadily toward the surface. Welcome this sensation with your total attention. Communicate to Shiva, "Yes, now, I'm coming!"

Shiva, watch carefully so you can learn the signs of a woman's sexual climax. For example, just before orgasm, Shakti's breathing may become shallow and her body may become very still, as if she is listening, waiting for the ultimate sensation to arise in her. This is because the sensations in her cleo become so pleasurable that chaotic bodily movements would distract her from experiencing their intensity. Or, alternatively, she may tense her thigh and leg muscles, raising her feet off the mattress.

As Shakti moves into orgasm, you will feel her cleo and vagina pulsing with a series of contractions. Her cleo will become so sensitive that it can be stimulated only very lightly or perhaps not at all.

After orgasm there will be a period, lasting anywhere from three to thirty minutes, when Shakti may not want you to touch this delicate trigger point.

Shiva, stay in communication with Shakti. After a few minutes have passed, ask her whether you can continue the massage. Sometimes, a woman's orgasm is composed of many miniorgasms that build on top of one another. The woman's first reaction may be "Okay, that's it, I've had my orgasm," but, with a little stimulation, she quickly realizes that she is ready to go on, opening herself to even more excitement.

STAGE 7: CLOSING THE SESSION GRACEFULLY

Shiva and Shakti, when either of you feels that the session is complete, gently ask your partner, "Is this a good time to make a pause?" or "I feel satisfied. Is it okay to stop?"

Phrase your suggestion as a question so that your partner feels included and respected. There has to be mutual agreement that it's time to close the session.

There is a simple ritual for ending the session that I call "closing the door."

Shiva, place your right hand on Shakti's heart center. Rest the palm of your left hand on Shakti's mound of Venus, with your fingers covering the lips of her Yoni, pressing slightly, helping Shakti's sexual energy flow back inside herself.

Look into each other's eyes for a few moments, then close your eyes, feeling how the energy that was focused on Shakti's cleo is now diffusing through both your bodies.

Five Basic Points of Clitoral Stimulation

Here are five basic points to remember for clitoral stimulation:

1. Erotic foreplay

2. Mastering the strokes

3. Rhythmic stimulation

4. Building arousal in steps

5. Eliciting full orgasm

Pointers

ACKNOWLEDGING SHIVA

Shakti, at the end of the session it's very important that you acknowledge Shiva and reward him for having done such a good job. Show him your gratitude and appreciation. Shower him with compliments, hugs, and, if it feels right, honor him with the ultimate reward of making love.

Remember, in this exercise, the man often becomes as vulnerable as the woman. He is like a new musician, learning to play Shakti's erotic instrument, discovering how to bring forth the right notes of orgasmic pleasure. He will want to be reassured that his audience has appreciated the concert.

PERSISTENCE PAYS OFF

Shiva, exploring all the strokes available for clitoral stimulation may take up to three sessions, so don't be in a hurry to "get it." Acquiring this new skill is bound to take time.

In the beginning, a certain patience and stamina is required. You must be prepared to "be in it for the long haul," giving pleasure to Shakti in a steady, supportive way so that she can relax, trust, move through any resistance, and reach a point where she can fully enjoy her orgasmic pleasure.

Shakti, you are the one who decides how long you want the stimulation to continue. You know when Shiva has attained mastery when he is as skillful at giving you a clitoral orgasm as you are at giving one to yourself. At this stage, you can totally relax into his expert hands.

Shiva, when you stimulate Shakti's cleo you may feel that your fingers are becoming delicate antennae that not only give but also receive pleasure. You may feel Shakti's warm, fiery energy flowing into you, turning you on, giving you an erection. This can be a very beautiful experience.

However, giving a clitoral massage can also be a bit of a technical task for you, so be patient and your persistence will pay off.

PRESENCE AND PLEASURE

Shakti, there are times when communicating with Shiva will be difficult. This can happen when you get lost in pleasure, when you are experiencing resistance, or when a particular thought or idea captures your attention and distracts you from the exercise.

Shiva, you can learn how to "read" Shakti, noticing when she becomes silent, when she no longer seems to be present, or when her pelvis becomes still or starts to pull way from your fingers.

If Shakti doesn't say anything, gently ask her a question, such as "How does this feel?"

Use as few words as possible. Getting into a conversation may distract both of you from the exercise, cutting the flow of sexual energy. For example, a question like "What's going on?" invites a long explanation. It is better to ask simple, specific questions like "Does this feel good?" "Do you want more?" "Shall I press more firmly?"

The eternal feminine draws us upward.

—GOETHE

Shakti, the key to good sexual communication is always to address what you like first, before you ask for a change. For example, "This is good, but now I'd like to try . . ." rather than saying "Hey, this doesn't feel good." In this way you acknowledge that Shiva is open and available to you and that critical feedback is likely to discourage him. By staying positive, his willingness to give is respected.

Watch how the mind takes you away from ecstasy. For example, you're feeling relaxed, enjoying the stimulation, and then suddenly you're thinking of the kids at school or the groceries to buy for supper . . . Before you know it, you're not feeling anything. You have detached yourself from your sensations.

Catch yourself when this happens and come back to the present. Here's a great tip: exhale all the way out, bringing your attention fully to your Yoni as you do so, holding a vivid picture of it in your mind (as described in chapter 3), visualizing that you are pushing all your energy down into your Yoni, seeing your blood flowing into your cleo and your vaginal lips. Immediately you will start to feel more. This is a real key for enhancing female pleasure.

Primordial all-accommodating spaciousness is the fundamental quality of the feminine.

—JOSÉ ARGUELLES

BEGINNER'S MIND: EMPTY CUP

Shiva, be careful not to enter a session with preconceived ideas about what Shakti wants, how she will behave, what goal has to be attained, or that you have to deliver the ultimate cosmic orgasm in the next thirty minutes. Shakti, the same applies to you.

In my experience, people often come to this exercise with all kinds of expectations, and this results in unnecessary disappointment when something entirely different occurs.

Come to each session with a fresh mind, like a beginner, like an empty cup that is about to be filled with unknown things. There is no need to know what is going to happen. There is no need to perform. Be open to whatever sensations and experiences arise. The more relaxed and easy you are, the better it gets.

CONTAINING SEXUAL AROUSAL

Shakti, once you have the ability to move easily into orgasm, a new and exciting dimension can be added to the exercise. Now you can allow Shiva to determine the length of the session, stopping when he feels tired or no longer comfortable.

This creates a challenge for you, because you may be left in a condition of strong sexual arousal without orgasmic release, feeling very turned on, wanting more yet not receiving it.

Your challenge is to relax into your sexual energy, allowing it to be absorbed in your body. This is not easy but is an important stage in building a strong orgasmic charge. It can also be a delightful sensation in itself.

Two partners in sexual magic, Laura and Ted, describe the difficulties and rewards of this stage. They had been practicing clitoral stimulation for about two weeks, with many sessions ending in full clitoral orgasm. Then, as Laura recalls:

> One night, Ted stopped about fifteen minutes after we had started, saying he was feeling tired and didn't have energy to go on. It was at a point when I was really getting into it,

when my excitement was rising toward my first strong peak.

Even though we'd agreed that Ted could determine the timing, I had a strong impulse to say "No, wait, you can't do this. You can't leave me like this." But then I thought, "Well, why not just follow the exercise and see what happens?"

As I got up from the couch, I could feel my pussy pulsing with energy, with desire. Ted headed for the bathroom to have a shower and prepare for bed, but I found myself walking restlessly around the house in this stage of great sexual excitement. I felt more horny than at any time in my life, because for two weeks we'd been practicing this massage and I'd been having a great time.

After a while, I figured I'd just go to Ted and ask him to finish me off, but then I started feeling awkward, almost like some sort of cheap slut who has to beg for sex, so I didn't. Instead, I started feeling angry with him, thinking "what kind of uncaring creep leaves a woman like this?"

Then I started laughing, because suddenly I knew how guys must feel when they are all charged up with excitement, ready to burst, and the girlfriend just kisses them on the cheek and says good night. My clitoris was aching at that moment, just wanting release in sexual climax.

Feminine wisdom accords with no abstract, unrelated code of law by which dead stars or atoms circulate in empty space. It is a wisdom that is bound and stays to the earth, to organic growth. Matriarchal consciousness is the wisdom of the earth.

—ERICH NEUMANN

I thought about pleasuring myself, but I wanted to see where the energy would go if I just stayed with the feeling, not doing anything about it. I heard Ted get into bed, and then there was silence in the house.

I turned off the downstairs lights and slid out of my bathrobe, then opened the curtains so I could see the city lights. After a while, I started wandering slowly from room to room, with no clothes on, softly touching my body now and then. As much as I could, I relaxed into the throbbing feelings in my sex. I gave in to the situation, giving myself permission to be this way.

Gradually, I noticed a kind of sensuousness spreading through my body, a delicious, silky feeling that wasn't localized in my pussy but all over me. I picked up a silk scarf and begin to play with it, slowly drawing it across my body, around my neck, down my legs. It felt cool and soft on my skin. I was being filled with pleasure in a different way, not so direct, more exquisite. Everything I touched had a sensual quality to it, the smoothness of the tabletop, the fine lace of the curtains, the softness of the carpet . . .

After a while, I no longer wanted sexual release. I still felt sexual—extremely sexual, very erotic—but I didn't want to do anything about it. I was really enjoying this new feeling. This went on for a couple of hours, then I began to feel tired and went to bed. When I saw Ted lying there, curled up, fast asleep, I felt grateful to him, that he'd been too tired to go on, otherwise I wouldn't have had this extraordinary experience. I went to sleep feeling very happy and content.

Laura's experience is indicative of the way sexual energy can be transformed. The clitoris is the most *yang* part of the female organ. In other words, it has male qualities. When aroused, it can be very demanding, pulling you toward climax with the feeling "I've got to do something about this right now!"

Women, this is how men usually feel when sexually aroused, so enjoy this opportunity of deepening your understanding of your partner's biological urges. In this stage of the exercise, the trick is to stay on the edge of your desire without wanting to get anywhere. Then the energy can move in a totally new direction.

OVERCOMING SEXUAL SABOTAGE

As I already mentioned, when it comes to allowing ourselves sexual pleasure, a surprising number of us women don't believe we deserve it.

In the theater of our childhood years, many of us were trained to follow a script in which Daddy played the leading role and our parts were "walk-ons" as supporting cast. We always had to do something, give something,

We are bearers of magic and our circle of support is a circle of mystical power. It is a woman's prerogative to know of magic and to practice and to use her knowledge to help the world.

—MARIANNE WILLIAMSON

serve someone in order to value our role in the drama. Hence, we have difficulty in feeling that we deserve pleasure, that we can just lie down and receive.

In addition, many women today have cultivated a dynamic male aspect to their personalities in order to compete as men's equals in a world that is still essentially patriarchal. This can make it difficult for us to switch gears, to become soft, open, vulnerable, and receptive.

These difficulties often manifest themselves in a variety of strategies designed to sabotage those situations in which we receive sexual satisfaction.

For example, Renee, an educational therapist in her mid-thirties and a student of sexual magic, had no difficulty learning the practices outlined here. But when she began to receive clitoral stimulation from her partner, everything changed.

Renee explains:

> I had a lot of trouble keeping my agreement with Mike, my partner, that I would receive a "do" once a day between two and three in the afternoon. That was the time that worked best for us, but, even though I'm self-employed and schedule my own hours, I felt guilty about leaving work to go lie down and prepare for orgasm.
>
> One way or another, I ended up not arriving on

time, or found myself talking on the phone until the last minute before joining Mike so that I wasn't really in the mood, or I'd try to pick a fight just before the session, or I'd have a headache, until Mike finally sat me down and said, "Renee, what's going on here? It's like you're doing me a big favor by coming to these sessions, but you're the one who's receiving!"

At first, I tried to deny what was going on, but Mike just kept pointing out what was happening and pretty soon I had to admit that it was true. After that, I paid more attention to the things I did before a session, and even though I still went through feelings of guilt, or worrying that I couldn't spare the time, I made sure that I arrived at the sessions on time and gave myself fully to the experience.

Even so, I still noticed a moment of discomfort, right when I had to lie down and spread my legs. It was like giving up control over my most private part. I also noticed feelings of shame, feeling somehow cheap that I could just walk in, take off my clothes, and lie down, exposing myself like this. But then I would say to myself, "The hell with it. This is for me. I don't care if it's ladylike or not—it feels great!"

An hour and a half later I would go back to my office, orgasmic, and happy, seeing everything with fresh eyes. It was clear that the work issues I'd been worrying about were no big deal. I'd exaggerated them to justify not giving myself the sessions. Moreover, some of my clients started commenting on how good I looked, and from then on I could keep a more relaxed attitude.

I remember one session, particularly, that was a breakthrough for me. We'd spent a long time finding a stroke I really liked and then Mike settled into a steady rhythm that seemed to go on forever. During this time, I went through so many fears, like "This is not for me; I'll never manage; I can't do it; I'm not really an orgasmic person; I'm taking too long; he's getting bored . . ."

But Mike just stayed with the massage in a steady, relaxed way, giving me reassurance until, in the end, I finally let go and had the most extraordinary orgasm of my life. It was a real teaching in how not to sell myself short and also gave me a tremendous trust in Mike, my partner.

After becoming familiar with the various ways of inducing a clitoral orgasm, the next step is to explore the G-Spot.

EXERCISE: PLEASURING THE GODDESS SPOT (THE G-SPOT)

Purpose and benefits
Through this exercise, you will discover the pleasure available to Shakti through massaging and stimulating her G-

Spot. Massage of the G–Spot will heal any negative or painful sensations that may be connected to this part of the Yoni, allowing Shakti to broaden her spectrum of sexual pleasure and facilitate her experience of vaginal orgasm.

This session can be done as a continuation of the previous exercise, or separately.

Preparations

- ☙ Shiva also creates the Magic Circle to welcome Shakti in an atmosphere of sensuality and security.

- ☙ Shakti pampers herself in readiness to relax and enjoy.

- ☙ Remember to have some water or fruit juice handy to quench your thirst, and be sure that the room is warm enough to work comfortably without clothing.

- ☙ As with the clitoral massage, Shiva listens and supports, while Shakti guides and receives.

- ☙ The best lubricants for massaging inside the vagina are water based, such as Astroglide or K–Y Jelly. Oil-based lubricants tend to clog the pores of the vaginal canal, preventing natural lubrication.

- ☙ Shiva, remember to have clean, trim, smooth nails.

- Shakti, make sure your bladder is empty.

- Allow sixty to ninety minutes for this exercise.

Practice

STAGE 1: SENSUAL FOREPLAY WITH THE CLITORIS

Shiva, invite Shakti into the Magic Circle. Help her to lie in the same basic posture that was described for clitoral massage.

For the massage of Shakti's G-Spot you may wish to sit directly between her legs, or you may prefer the position you used for clitoral stimulation. Experience will show you which is best.

Make sure that you have enough pillows under your forearms to support their weight so that your hands don't get tired. Have both kinds of lubricant near at hand, the oil-based lubricant for Shakti's cleo and the water based for her Goddess Spot.

Tune in to your partner. Put one hand on Shakti's heart center and the other on her Yoni. Synchronize your breathing. Look into her eyes, feeling the bond of love, acceptance, and compassion that connects you in this sacred experiment. Let everything except this precious moment fall away from your mind; forget any preoccupations or concerns.

Shiva, caress Shakti's body, taking plenty of time.

The more Shakti is aroused through this delicate foreplay, the easier it will be for her to receive pleasure.

Using plenty of lubricant, caress Shakti's Yoni, beginning with the outer lips, then spreading the lips apart and circling the vaginal canal. When you feel Shakti is ready, focus on her clitoris, playing with a variety of strokes, then settling into a slow, steady, rhythmic stroke that gives her pleasure.

STAGE 2: APPROACHING THE GODDESS SPOT

Shiva, as you stimulate the cleo, let your free hand slide between her legs, under her sacrum, with your thumb pressed lightly against the opening of her vaginal canal.

Take time to bring Shakti to a level of strong clitoral excitement. As she becomes more and more aroused, your thumb will be gradually sucked inside by a series of pulsations, or contractions of her Yoni. Shakti's Yoni is welcoming your thumb like a penis.

The connection between your thumb and Shakti's Yoni can help you "read" her level of excitement. When the tissues around her vagina become engorged and swollen, when she is lubricating, when her pelvis pushes forward as if wanting to swallow your thumb, she is ready for you to begin stimulating her G-Spot.

Ask Shakti, "May I visit you?" If her answer is "yes," gently and slowly slide your thumb out of Shakti's Yoni. Now you are going to penetrate with the index and middle finger of the same hand.

The palm of your hand is facing upward and your two fingers are slightly curved, or crooked, so that, once inside, they can press against the roof of Shakti's Yoni at the "twelve o'clock" position.

Be sure that your fingers are well lubricated with a water-based lubricant before entering.

As you penetrate Shakti's Yoni, continue to massage her cleo lightly with your other hand.

STAGE 3: FINDING THE GODDESS SPOT

The G-Spot is felt as a bumplike place, the size of a pea, on the roof of the vaginal canal, beneath the pubic bone. Here, the tissues have a raspy quality, rather like the tongue of a cat, differing from the smoothness of the surrounding vaginal wall. You will need to probe the area, pressing fairly strongly, until Shakti experiences a specifically sensitive point.

Shakti, if you have never been stimulated in this area before, pressure from Shiva's fingers may manifest itself as a feeling of burning or a sharp nerve reaction like a

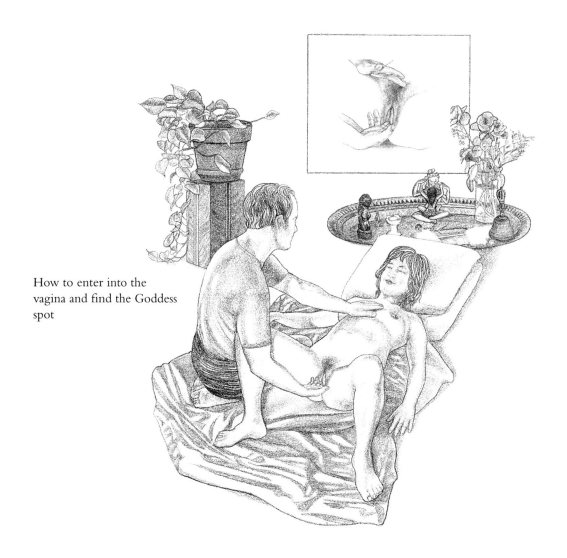

How to enter into the
vagina and find the Goddess
spot

"zing" that passes through the area of your Yoni. In other words, you may not feel pleasant sensations the first few times your G-Spot is touched. On the other hand, you may immediately feel a warm glow of pleasure, or you may feel nothing special.

If you feel the need to urinate, remember that this is probably an illusion caused by the nerve connection with your bladder, which you emptied before this exercise. If possible, stay with the session rather than breaking off to go to the bathroom.

It's important not to get discouraged by feelings of discomfort in your G-Spot. Like any part of your body that hasn't been touched for a long time, there are likely to be a few aches and pains as tensions start to release.

Shiva, when you have found the G-Spot, remove your other hand from Shakti's cleo and rest it on her belly. She needs to be able to experience her G-Spot free from other stimulation.

Shakti, it is usually helpful for you to move while Shiva is stimulating your G-Spot. Rock your pelvis, do the PC Pump, breathe strongly, and use your voice to sigh and moan, relaxing your throat and neck.

Remember: The Three Keys to enhancing your feelings and physical sensations are breathing, movement, and sound.

STAGE 4: STROKES FOR PLEASURING THE GODDESS SPOT

Shiva, you may have to press quite deeply, more deeply than you would expect, before your partner feels something. There are three basic strokes for G-Spot stimulation, using the two fingers that are inside Shakti's Yoni. Begin to experiment, checking which gives her most pleasure.

1. Massage in a zigzag pattern, moving crossways over the whole area. This will relax the G-Spot and the surrounding tissues.

2. Massage in and out, your fingers running over the roof of Shakti's vagina from the opening to the cervix. This way, your fingers pass over the G-Spot without staying on it.

3. Place two fingers directly on the G-Spot and begin to pulsate, pressing strongly in this area.

Shakti, the degree of pressure is up to you. You are the guide. Make sure you give Shiva plenty of feedback.

Shiva, try different strokes and pressures. Circle around the G-Spot. Pulse on the same spot. Stroke in and out.

STAGE 5: GENERATING AROUSAL

Shiva, you know you have found the right stroke and rhythm when Shakti gets the glorious feeling that she is making love with your fingers. Her pelvis will lift up and she will get into a rhythmic movement with her hips, as if she is being penetrated by your penis.

Shakti, communicate what you really want. You can say things like "Yes, yes, that's it, keep going," or "Oh yes, this is good, do it to me, give it to me!" It can be very enjoyable to call for your pleasure in this uninhibited way.

Shiva, this is a signal for you to stroke Shakti's G-Spot in a rhythmic way, helping her climb toward new heights of sexual pleasure. However, be prepared for unexpected changes. On the G-Spot, a certain stroke can provide great pleasure one moment and the next moment can suddenly cease to be stimulating.

Shakti, if this happens, don't hesitate to request a change. Shiva, follow your partner's guidance.

Shiva, use your free hand to press on the G-Spot from outside the Yoni, on Shakti's lower belly. This is a good way to enhance G-Spot sensation. Another way is to rub her lower belly and the area of her ovaries.

Shakti, allow the sensations to expand through your pelvic area and your body. You can help to spread the energy by massaging your breasts and other regions that feel sensual and erotic.

She is the primordial Shakti. She is the supreme, whose nature is unoriginated and undisturbed joy. She is eternally utterly incomparable, the sea of all that moves or is motionless, the spotless mirror in which is revealed the radiant form of Shiva.

—KAMA KALA VISLASA SUTRA

56

Stage 6: Orgasm of the Goddess Spot

Shakti, don't feel that you need to have a G-Spot orgasm, or vaginal orgasm, as this may create unnecessary tension and disappointment. In this session, you are getting to know your G-Spot and its response to stimulation.

However, if you do come close to orgasm, you will find that you need a lighter touch on your G-Spot. Communicate this to your beloved. The more the excitement, the less stimulation.

Continued light stimulation can bring a strong vaginal orgasm, with contractions deep inside your vaginal canal. There may be a release of ejaculatory fluid from tiny glands near your urethra. Relax and let it happen. These sensations can last one minute or five, perhaps even longer.

Shakti, continue receiving G-Spot stimulation until your appetite for sexual pleasure is satiated.

Acknowledge Shiva's generous contribution to your sexual awakening.

Close the session with a Heart Salutation.

Five Stages of G-Spot Stimulation

Here are five basic points to remember for stimulating the G-Spot:

1. Erotic foreplay

2. Stimulating the cleo

3. Finding the G-Spot

4. Mastering the strokes

5. Building arousal

Pointers

MOVING THROUGH LAYERS

Shakti, if you feel there is a lot of tension in the area of your G-Spot, or a sense of pain or burning, then keep the first session fairly short, say five minutes, or until you want to stop. Feel free to progress in stages that feel comfortable.

You may go through many layers of sensations in your G-Spot, some tense, some pleasurable. You may require three to four sessions before this spot becomes sensitive to pleasure.

Remember, female responses vary widely. Some women experience pleasure right away, some never feel anything special, while some discover other areas inside the vagina that are pleasurable when stimulated. I have discovered several such places, especially along the roof of the vaginal canal, on the same line as the G–Spot, between the opening and the cervix.

JUMP INTO THE UNKNOWN

As I mentioned in the previous exercise, one of the biggest barriers to sexual pleasure is expectation. People tend to bring certain ideas to a particular exercise and, when reality does not match this expectation, they feel they have failed.

This is a misunderstanding. In my experience, there is always a deep teaching in each session, regardless of how it goes. The best approach is to come to each session totally fresh, not knowing what is going to happen. I am giving you a basic road map, but there are many delightful detours to be explored. You are moving into unknown territory.

EXERCISE: ALCHEMY OF THE BLENDED FEMALE ORGASM

Purpose and benefits

To give a woman the ultimate experience of prolonged sexual orgasm, blending the stimulation of her two principle pleasure spots in a subtle and ever-expanding orgasmic response.

Preparation

- ❦ Shiva, prepare the Magic Circle and create a beautiful atmosphere in the room. Check that you have plenty of lubricants handy and also a jug of water.

- ❦ Shakti, take a long, luxurious shower or bath, using your favorite oils, pampering yourself.

- ❦ Allow sixty to ninety minutes for this exercise.

Practice

STAGE 1: ENTERING THE GARDEN

Shiva, lead Shakti into the Magic Circle and help her to lie in a comfortable position.

When you are both settled, begin foreplay, lightly caressing Shakti's body, teasing and pleasuring her Yoni, gradually focusing on her cleo.

When Shakti is ready, begin to stimulate her cleo with a stroke that feels just right.

Let the index and middle fingers of your free hand rest at the door of Shakti's Yoni. Don't be in a hurry to enter. Wait at the door and let Shakti's arousal increase until your fingers are drawn inside her Yoni with a pulsating, sucking motion. This is the right moment to ask her

"May I come in?" or, if you wish to be more poetic, "May I enter your sacred garden?"

Begin G-Spot stimulation. Find the best finger position, looking for the right pressure and stroke on her G-Spot.

Establish a rhythm of stimulating the G-Spot and the clitoris at the same time. Or, if Shakti prefers, you can alternate between the two.

STAGE 2: DOUBLE ACTION STROKES
Shiva, there are three basic strokes for stimulating Shakti toward a blended orgasm:

1. Leave your fingers anchored on her G-Spot, with little or no movement, while rhythmically stimulating her cleo.

2. Leave your fingers anchored on her cleo, with little or no movement, while vigorously stimulating her G-Spot.

3. Create a rhythmic, blended movement in both places. For example, you can run your fingers over her cleo down toward the mouth of her Yoni, while your fingers on her G-Spot push inward. In this way, the hands move in opposite directions, as if going toward each other, in a kind of double-action massage.

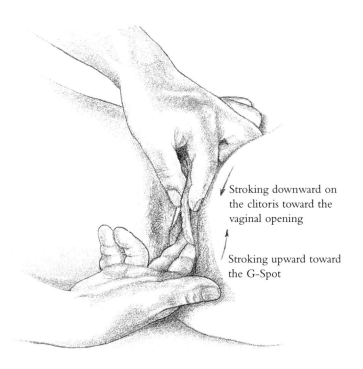

Double action strokes: pleasuring the clitoris emphasizing the downward movements; stimulating the G-Spot emphasizing the upward movement

Stroking downward on the clitoris toward the vaginal opening

Stroking upward toward the G-Spot

Or you can grip the shaft of Shakti's cleo with two fingers and stimulate the tip with a third finger, while the fingers of your other hand run in and out over her G-Spot.

There are many subtle variations to be explored as you learn to pleasure Shakti skillfully with combined strokes. It is as if the fingers of your two hands are having a dialogue with each other.

Shakti, it is your job to guide Shiva, saying how you

want it, what combination works best, and when you want to explore a new variation. Good communication is essential to finding the right strokes. Remember to stay positive: "Yes, I like that. Now try this . . ."

STAGE 3: EXPANDING ORGASM

Once you have found the best combination of strokes, let Shiva know so that he can continue the same rhythm for a long time. You need regular stimulation so that you can relax and build slowly toward orgasm.

Shiva, the more intense Shakti's excitement becomes, the more regular your strokes need to be. When your partner seems to be coming close to climax, slow down, tease, give her the promise but keep her waiting. Build her arousal in steps, bringing her several times to a peak without going over the edge.

G stands for Growth, Good, Glorious, Goddess. Find the G spot, and you've found your way home.

—DR. ZANGPO

Shakti, you can generate a really exciting sensation that keeps spreading inside and out, like ripples that keep expanding until they cover your whole pond. Your body is moving deeper and deeper into relaxation, while your sexual excitement builds higher and higher.

Remember to use the Three Keys and the PC Pump to help enhance and spread your orgasmic sensations.

Your first orgasm is likely to be explosive, with pulsing contractions inside your Yoni and a great release of energy throughout your pelvic area. Afterward, it's possible to go on. You can have several orgasms, so it's important for Shiva to keep his hands in place, not moving, while the orgasm happens.

STAGE 4: INVOLUNTARY STREAMING SENSATIONS

Shiva, when Shakti's first orgasm has passed, slowly begin to stimulate the cleo and G-Spot once more, building toward even higher peaks of pleasure.

Shakti, now your orgasmic sensations are likely to be more subtle, like energy streaming, like a current of pleasurable feeling that keeps circulating and pulsing inside your pelvis and perhaps through other areas of your body. You are not doing anything. It is involuntary. It is happening to you.

You are entering an ecstatic state that is timeless, floating, deeply relaxed, and meditative, in which your body is so sensitive that very little stimulation is required. This can continue for as long as you wish.

One group participant described this state as follows:

> I had this incredible surprise: the orgasm was going on by itself. I had the impression of having tuned in to a new frequency of pleasure, as if ecstasy is available to me all the time, but I didn't know where to turn the dial to find the right wavelength.

When the session ended, the sensations continued. I slowly tried to get up, always watching whether they would disappear. They didn't, so I started to whirl slowly, like a Sufi, turning on the spot with my arms held high.

I had the impression that my orgasm was rising and falling up and down my body, from my feet all the way to my head, and through me from the center of the earth all the way to the stars.

Five Stages of Blended Orgasm

Here are five points to remember for creating a blended orgasm:

1. Stimulating the clitoris

2. Combined stimulation of the clitoris and G-Spot

3. Generating sexual arousal in steps

4. First orgasmic release

5. Ongoing, subtle sensations

Pointers

LETTING IT HAPPEN

In the beginning, good communication is required to find the right combination of strokes for stimulating the clitoris while simultaneously massaging the G-Spot. Later, it is helpful if Shakti can stop talking and simply relax, while

Shiva maintains a steady rhythm, so that she can become completely receptive to this exquisite experience.

For this to happen, both partners need to have thoroughly trained themselves in all the various aspects of clitoral and G-Spot stimulation. Then Shakti can lie back and let it happen.

QUICKER ORGASMIC RESPONSE

One of the great advantages of this practice is that it is an excellent preparation for normal lovemaking. After experiencing blended orgasm, most women are able to enjoy much quicker orgasmic response during penetration with a penis.

Moreover, research has shown that expanding orgasm in this way balances the left and right hemispheres of the brain and enhances the production of endorphins, making people more relaxed, healthy, and happy, re ducing tension and stress. This, surely, is magic in itself!

The Easy Approach to Orgasm

After practicing these methods of expanding orgasm for many years and learning how to integrate these wonderful experiences in my love life, I realize that my approach is somewhat different from other experts in the field.

For example, in their book *ESO*, Alan and Donna Brauer describe a three-level orgasm for women. The first level is characterized by rhythmic squeezing and relaxing pulsations around the entry of the vagina. The second involves involuntary contractions, pushing outwards, in the deeper part of the vagina and around the uterus. The third is a continuous stream of pleasure within the vaginal canal that happens effortlessly and which may continue for up to thirty minutes.

In my experience, orgasms do not necessarily follow a logical continuum from one step to the next. Each one has its own unique flavor, and I don't wish to create performance anxiety in my readers by saying "This is how it has to be."

Certainly, the Brauers' research is very valuable, opening up new fields of sexual understanding, but your attention needs to be focused on generating the maximum amount of orgasmic power as easily and as comfortably as possible.

I love being female. I love being with a man. If I ground my sexual energy, I am here and now, otherwise I'm just roaming. Grounded sexual energy brings peace and nourishment to the soul.

—A Tantrika's Diary

It doesn't really matter how it happens. Whether your orgasm has three stages, one, or four is not so relevant. The real point is for you, the woman, to be able to have beautiful expanded orgasmic responses that are pleasurable and intense, free from pain or tension.

These responses may last a few seconds, a few minutes, or half an hour, but duration of the orgasm is not the goal. The goal is for each individual woman to discover, with the help of her partner, all the orgasmic secrets hidden in her body and to unlock them one by one, in her own style.

Not only is this a magical experience in itself, it is also a very powerful aid to sexual magic, as we shall see later in the book. However, first we must focus on Shiva and the orgasmic pleasures that can be made available to him, for he has done well in honoring and pleasuring Shakti, and it is time for him to be suitably rewarded.

SHIVA'S MAGIC:
The Alchemy of Male Orgasm

Men, you are about to enter what I consider the greatest adventure in which you can become involved—greater than Columbus's discovery of the Americas, greater than conquering Mount Everest or landing on the moon. It is the adventure that consists in discovering, honoring, and cultivating the magical power contained in your Vajra—literally "thunderbolt"—your male sexual organ.

This power, when fully engaged, brings virility, dominion, and enchantment into your love life and a deep sense of kingliness to your being. Good lovers are the natural emperors of this world, for they are rooted in their manhood, at ease with themselves, and greatly loved and appreciated by their female partners.

Since ancient times the Vajra has been worshiped as a symbol of the fertility through which the earth grows new crops, through which herds multiply, through which the tribe feeds itself, prospers, and grows strong. Although this celebration of male sexual power may be difficult for a modern Western man to believe, it's true. Although many of today's men feel attacked simply for being men, it hasn't always been that way. You deserve your own special hymn, a "hymn to the Vajra," so relax and enjoy yourself while I sing a few verses for you.

Each spring, in Japan, your manhood is represented in large sculptures, blown up to gigantic proportions—a truly cosmic erection—and is paraded through city streets to celebrate the gods of fertility and renewal, with, of course, much song, wine, and sake. Dionysius, the drunken Greek god of ecstasy, also embodies phallic energy, helping people to dance, celebrate, abandon the rigid formalities of society for a while and let go into an uninhibited, orgiastic, and ecstatic state.

In Northern Europe, the horned god Pan, half goat and half man, is portrayed as a smiling, laughing deity who reigns over nature and the animal kingdom, walking around with a big erection, symbolizing constant enjoyment, a being who is always ready for sexual action.

These mythological beings represent dynamic energies that are part of you. They represent your own phallic strength and the qualities that exude from it such as manhood, power, potency, virility, creativity, courage, decisiveness, action, the ability to have a handle on events, to shape and control powerful forces.

If this eulogy sounds too good to be true, it is only because men are currently passing through a period of confusion about their role in relationship to women. Having acknowledged, to some extent, a brutish past in which they dominated and exploited women, many men are now trying to demonstrate that they can be as soft, gentle, and sensitive as their love partners.

Imagine their surprise, therefore, when they discover that women don't really want this newfangled masculinity—at least, not at the cost of losing the male strength they so much appreciate. True, they don't want to be dominated by aggressive and controlling male patriarchs, but neither do they want men to be so concerned about pleasing women that they lose their own sense of identity, strength, and purpose.

Small wonder, then, that today's male is a somewhat perplexed and angry creature. He can be forgiven for

All thoughts, all passions, all
  delights,
Whatever stirs this mortal
  frame,
All are but ministers of Love,
And feed his sacred flame.

—SAMUEL TAYLOR COLERIDGE
Love

A traditional phallic symbol in India, representing the qingham (penis) inserted in the yoni (vagina)

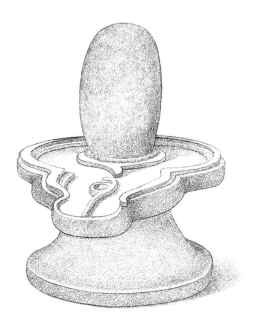

throwing up his hands in despair and saying "Okay, I give up! What the hell am I supposed to be, hard or soft, dominant or passive, masculine or feminine?" Then, before receiving a reply, he disappears into the local branch of the men's movement to share his woes with like-minded casualties of the "new sexuality" of the nineties.

NATURAL MALE ENERGY

In answer to this dilemma, men, I have some good news for you. For a great many women—perhaps all women, in their heart of hearts—there is nothing more beautiful, exciting, and delicious than a man who is grounded in his sexuality, a man who is rooted in his virile, potent, natural male energy.

However, it is important to understand that when I use the phrase "natural male energy" I am referring to a very different phenomenon than the *machismo* that has been accepted as manhood in the past. Natural maleness is not to be attained, for example, through popping steroids to gain a muscular torso, or through doing push-ups on a woman for half an hour without coming, or through acquiring a cool, casual image by cutting yourself off from your feelings. These are symptoms of unnatural maleness, of an acquired facade, a chauvinistic mask, a stereotyped *macho* image that is a sexual fraud.

The reason that so many men choose to cultivate such a façade lies in a deep-seated conflict between biology and society, between lust and law, between animal energy and civilized ideals. It is worth taking a look at these conflicting forces to see the dynamic in which our luckless heroes have been caught.

The biological force puts men in the same category as any pack of healthy male animals: hanging out in fraternal groups, horsing around, butting each other, testing each other's strength, feeling horny when the rutting season begins, and then beating each other up to see who gets first privileges with the patiently waiting females.

However, the rules of conventional society say that such animalistic behavior is, well, *animalistic,* and therefore unworthy of the civilized male. It also says that male sexual feelings must be strictly controlled and mostly repressed, especially during those seemingly endless years of adolescence when young men's bodies are full of raging hormones that demand intense sexual activity.

Further, the rules clearly state that men may act out their animal competitiveness only in certain specifically allocated theaters, such as the football field, Wall Street, and the occasional war. Otherwise they must hold back their instinctual energies and behave with social politeness and decorum, especially in the company of women.

One cannot be strong without love. For love is not an irrelevant emotion; it is the blood of life, the power of reunion of the separated.

—PAUL TILLICH
The Eternal Now

This combination of seemingly contradictory forces, the animal and the social, has created a type of mutant maleness that is unique in the animal kingdom. The human male is supposed to look like a man, act like a man, but not behave like one. Not only must he repress his sexual and aggressive urges, he should, in addition, cultivate other unnatural qualities such as never showing fear, even when fear is an appropriate response, and never revealing any "weakness" such as weeping or feeling sad or helpless. Moreover, he should always be in command of himself and the situation around him.

Not surprisingly, this artificial condition has left men in a state of suspended animation, ready for action but usually not getting it, exhibiting their manliness and sexual potency yet rarely experiencing it as their personal reality. For too many men, the sexual climax is more like a sneeze, a sudden release of pent-up tension. The pleasure available to both man and woman is far shorter than it can or should be. That is why statistics show the average male orgasm lasts from two to ten seconds and occurs five to ten minutes after he begins to be excited. There is little opportunity for sexual magic in such an abrupt and speedy ejaculation.

In addition, man now has to deal with a feminist backlash to his long years of patriarchal rule. In the current war between the sexes, he is portrayed as the bad guy, the evildoer, the one who prowls around in the guise of a civilized human being, complete with suit and tie, but who is loaded with all kinds of dangerous hormones and nasty impulses that make him a potential sex maniac filled with a blind, unconscious lust that at a moment's notice can turn any woman into his helpless victim.

DRIVEN TO POWER IN ORDER TO MATE?

While men have abused their power in the past, there is also an instinctive tendency in women to seek out, and mate with, those men who wield the most power.

As evidence, I refer to an intriguing global research project conducted by David M. Buss, a psychology professor at the University of Michigan at Ann Arbor. In his book *The Evolution of Desire,* Buss shows how, even today, the overwhelming majority of women around the world— spanning all nations and cultures—are still attracted to men who exude an aura of being able to take care of them, provide for them, protect and nourish them.

Why would women seek powerful men? According to Professor Buss, the answer lies in our evolutionary psychology, in an instinct for survival that developed over thousands of years of living as nomadic hunter-gatherers in an untamed and frequently hostile environment. Under such primitive conditions, Buss argues, women naturally gravitated toward mates who could best protect and provide for them during pregnancy and early motherhood, when their self-sufficiency was inhibited by their infants.

Over time, this ancient but successful strategy became hard-wired into our psychology. As Buss points out, "If women over evolutionary history have preferred men who have resources and have the power and status to control those resources, then over time they will drive the evolution of status-seeking, power-seeking mechanisms in men."

In other words, by making power a criterion for mating, our sisters in earlier times were sending messages to their menfolk that they needed to be big, strong, wealthy, and in command of the situation. The men, eager to adopt any behavior likely to impress the fairer sex, responded to these messages by developing characteristics of being chauvinistic, autocratic, and overbearing.

Buss's conclusions are controversial, but from a lay viewpoint they seem to make sense, bringing a more balanced perspective to the issue of responsibility for centuries of inequality between the sexes—although I would find it loathsome if his theory were used to justify any kind of male supremacist ideology.

The real issue here is not who is to blame for the ugliness and sorrows of our past, but how to liberate ourselves from the limiting habits, beliefs, and ideas carried over from earlier times so that we can discover our true capacity for sexual fulfillment.

In an effort to restore the balance, many men these days are making Herculean efforts to satisfy their female partners sexually. Instead of leaping into the saddle for a quick ride in the grand urban-cowboy tradition, they are eager to satisfy a woman and are patiently and sensitively bringing their love partners to orgasmic climax before permitting themselves the ejaculatory release for which they yearn.

As a sexual being, man is still holding back, controlling and performing according to some socially acceptable ideal. The ideal may have expanded, so that now it includes satisfying the woman instead of ignoring her sexual needs. Yet men too can be multi-orgasmic.

INITIATION INTO THE NEW MANHOOD

In terms of sexual magic, it is essential that male sexual power be reclaimed, honored, and expanded, so that the alchemy of the combined orgasmic energy of a man and a woman who are entwined in deep Tantric embrace can happen at optimum power. The purpose of this chapter is to create a healthy, virile, male sexual energy that can meet the woman's energy in an ecstatic union, making powerful sexual magic.

Accomplishing this task is immensely enjoyable, and does not pressure the masculine ego to focus on sexual performance and achievement.

Rather, it lies in relaxation, in letting go, in allowing things to happen rather than forcing them to materialize on cue. To my male readers I would like to say: You have done enough; now it is your turn to lie back and receive.

In the following exercises, you will be invited to receive pleasure in a passive way, as your love partner stimulates first your penis, then your prostate gland, and then gives you a blended orgasm by stimulating both areas together. In this way, you will learn how to be deeply receptive, so that your sexual energy is not thrown outward in ejaculation but is absorbed inside your body, and your orgasmic capacity is expanded.

Through this exciting journey you have the chance to receive initiation into a new type of manhood, a new form of virility. This Tantric initiation may sometimes be difficult. It may take you through moments of not having an erection when you think you ought to have one, moments when you want to ejaculate and are being invited to keep the energy inside.

Raise your enjoyment to its highest power and then use it as spiritual rocket fuel.

—MAHA TANTRA ACANA

By mastering these challenges, you will come to experience a deeper sense of sexual potency. You will find yourself on an ascending curve of pleasure, rising to greater and greater heights of sexual fulfillment.

The most challenging part of this initiation into male sexual alchemy is to develop the inner strength that allows you to disassociate with your desire to ejaculate, your need to come, your impulse to release your sexual tension. The easier and more pleasurable part is to become receptive to an ever-widening pool of orgasmic energy that arises when your ejaculation is contained.

In the beginning you may feel that giving up your ejaculation, your familiar kind of genital orgasm, is no fun. You may get frustrated, even angry. It is an exercise in discipline, and you have to be willing to go through a period of delayed gratification in order to learn how to expand your sexual sensations, as you prepare for a whole-body orgasm instead of a localized genital one.

The payoff is going to be enormous, not only in the area of sexual magic but also in the field of normal love-making. Your new capacity to master your ejaculatory reflex means that you can decide when you finally want to let go, prolong your lovemaking ability, and satisfy your female partner fully as well as enjoy heightened orgasmic sensations yourself.

THREE STAGES OF EXPANDING MALE ORGASM

The exercises for expanding male orgasm are divided into three stages.

Stage 1

The woman stimulates the man's Vajra, or penis, finding ways to bring him close to ejaculation, then stopping just before the point of no return, allowing the aroused sexual energy to spread through the man's body.

Stage 2

Stimulation of Vajra is combined with external stimulation of the prostate gland, by massaging the perineum area, helping the man to broaden his range of sexual sensations.

Stage 3

Stimulation of Vajra is combined with massage of the prostate directly and internally, leading to a longer and more powerful orgasm.

*

This three-stage process allows the man to expand his orgasmic capacity in a series of steps, climbing toward sexual peaks, stopping each time before ejaculation, relaxing into the feelings that have been awakened, then climbing toward new and higher peaks.

Eventually, he comes to a place where there is no ejaculation happening but there is a continuous stream of orgasmic pleasure running through his sexual organs, his pelvic area, and his whole body. When he finally chooses to allow ejaculation, it lasts much longer, with much more powerful orgasmic sensations.

Before we move into the exercises, it will be instructive to examine the anatomy of the male sexual organ.

ANATOMY OF MALE SEXUALITY

The Vajra, or penis, is a relatively simple mechanism. It has no bones and no muscles, being composed mainly of spongy tissues. When a man is sexually aroused these spongy tissues become engorged with blood, stiffening Vajra and transforming it into a wonderfully energized, potent instrument of pleasure.

In today's male, the Vajra comes in two distinct

styles: the unaltered model, complete with foreskin, or the circumcised version from which most or all of the foreskin has been removed. Both varieties have an equal capacity to satisfy sexually the owner and his beloved partner.

The shaft of the Vajra extends from the body just below the pubic mound and ends in a distinctive head or glans that looks rather like a smooth mushroom cap. Here, the texture of the surface changes as normal body skin gives way to the polished roundness of the head. The color of the head is usually several shades darker than the skin of the shaft beneath.

At the top of the head is a small opening that marks the end of the urethra, a small tube that carries the body's waste fluids from the kidneys to be expelled through the Vajra as urine. This tube also carries a mixture of fluid from the prostate gland and testicles, to be expelled through the Vajra as semen in sexual ejaculation.

On the underside of the penis, just below the point at which the skin of the shaft attaches to the head, there is a particularly sensitive area known as the frenulum. When correctly stimulated, this spot can be a great source of sexual pleasure and for this reason I like to think of it as the male equivalent of the cleo, or clitoris.

Below the Vajra lies the scrotal sac. This contains two oval-shaped testicles that manufacture sperm and the male hormone testosterone. The hormones are absorbed into the body, but the sperm are stored in special bags inside the scrotal sac known as epididymides.

When a man becomes sexually excited, the sperm travels up from the testicles through the vas deferens tube to the prostate gland. This small gland is shaped like a chestnut and sits inside the body, in the bowl of the pelvis, between the Vajra and the anus.

You can feel your prostate by pressing on the perineum point, halfway between your scrotal sac and your anus. You will feel a soft, spongy area. This is where your prostate is hidden. When your Vajra is erect your prostate feels like the root of your erection, as if it were part of the same organ. Anatomically, this is not so, but in terms of how it feels there is a definite connection between the two.

If the man's frenulum can be compared to the woman's clitoris, then his prostate gland can be compared to the G-Spot, because it offers deeper and more lasting sensations of sexual orgasm. Both these areas will be explored in the exercises that follow.

At the moment of sexual climax, muscular contrac-

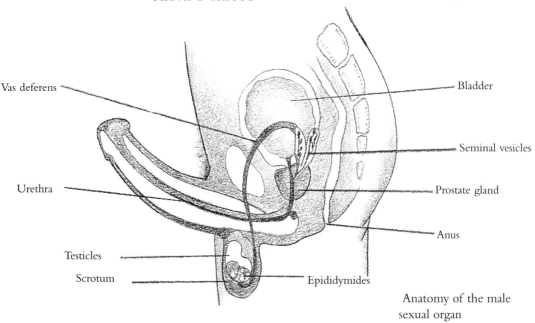

Vas deferens

Urethra

Testicles

Scrotum

Bladder

Seminal vesicles

Prostate gland

Anus

Epididymides

Anatomy of the male
sexual organ

tions around the prostate discharge a mixture of sperm
and prostatic fluid through the urethra and out of the
head of the Vajra.

EXERCISE: STIMULATING THE VAJRA

Purpose and benefits
Men, in the following exercises your love partner will be
pleasuring your sexual organ in new and delightful ways,
bringing you a whole new spectrum of sexual sensations

and expanding your orgasmic capacity. She will bring you close to ejaculation, then help you to relax and let this energy be absorbed in your body before moving again toward a new and higher peak.

For monogamous couples, here is a great opportunity to bring fresh excitement and depth to your sexual routine, varying roles and behavior that may have become fixed, boring, or dull. Now you can reawaken your enthusiasm and energy for each other as sexual partners, enhancing each other's pleasure a thousandfold.

This practice is also very suitable for—although certainly not limited to—men in their fifties, sixties, and seventies, because this kind of stimulation does not depend on having a full erection, nor does it involve the sexual athletics that are sometimes required during sexual intercourse, such as frequently changing body positions and supporting your weight on your arms, shoulders, or knees for long periods of time.

Shiva, the success of this wonderful session depends on your ability to become receptive, letting go of your traditional role as leader, initiator, and producer of sexual pleasure and experiencing instead the more feminine qualities of surrender, receptivity, and trust. However, you need to remain in charge as the one who leads and instructs

Shakti how to give you pleasure, guiding her actions, giving her continuous feedback on what she is doing.

Shakti, this exercise offers you a great opportunity to cultivate a sense of self-confidence and power. You are the cocreator, the equal partner, the giver, the provider of ecstasy. You will enjoy this exercise more if you understand that you are doing it for yourself, if you can say "Yes, I'm curious, excited . . . I want to learn how to master the art of giving a man pleasure . . . I want to know how his sexual organ responds . . . I want to see him moan with ecstasy at my touch . . . I want to feel my skills as a lover, as the one who initiates these feelings in him while remaining centered on myself."

However, be alert that you do not fall into the trap of overwhelming Shiva and taking control of the exercise, as this may inhibit his ability to express what he needs and fully experience his pleasure. Allow him to tell you how to stimulate the Vajra and follow his suggestions exactly.

Shiva and Shakti, the success of this exercise will depend on your ability to establish and maintain a nourishing heart connection with each other. I emphasize this because some couples may be tempted to skip over the early stages of the exercise in their eagerness to explore direct stimulation of the Vajra. But the initial steps, especially those bonding the two lovers through the heart, are of great help in paving the way for a successful session.

Preparations

- Stimulation and massage of the Vajra requires lots of good-quality lubricant. Water-based lubricants tend to dry faster than oil-based ones when applied externally. My personal preference is to use a pure, organic oil such as olive oil, which can be applied in abundance and has no harmful effect on the Vajra's delicate skin. It can also be used to massage other areas of the body. Alternatively, any good-quality organic massage oil will serve your purpose.

- Create a special code word for Shiva to use when he comes close to the point of ejaculation and wants Shakti to stop stimulating his Vajra. He can say "now" or "stop" to indicate the moment when Shakti should cease all stimulation.

- Shakti, this time you are the one who creates the Sacred Space for Shiva. Bring any objects that have a strong male connotation like drums, male sculptures, feathers, photos, phallic symbols, and so on. Create an intriguing atmosphere through incense, candles, and subtle lighting. You may also want to bring a humorous and appropriate toy, like a model of King

Kong. Be sure to wear something sexy, like a see-through blouse, or be naked except for a beautiful *lungi* around your hips and a flower in your hair. Whatever your choice, make sure your clothes allow your arms and torso to more freely.

🖎 Shiva, give yourself time to have a luxurious shower, cleaning yourself thoroughly, especially your genitals and anus. Put on your favorite cologne and prepare to be pampered by Shakti. Make sure that your bladder is empty.

🖎 Shakti, check that your fingernails are trimmed and smooth.

🖎 Allow sixty to ninety minutes for this exercise, making sure there will be no interruptions.

STAGE 1: MEETING THROUGH THE HEART
Shakti, bring Shiva into the sacred space. Help him to feel welcome, relaxed, and at home. You may want to dance energetically together for a few minutes, to rid yourselves of any tension.

Enjoy a long Melting Hug. Breathe deeply, in synchronicity together as you do so.

Sit facing each other on cushions.

Shakti, place your right hand on Shiva's heart, then

take his right hand and put it on your own heart. Gaze softly into each other's eyes, harmonizing your breathing, listening for each other's heartbeat. Breathe slowly and deeply. Feel the love and trust that is flowing between you as your embark on this new and exciting adventure.

Shakti, dip your fingers in some special oil or perfume and bless Shiva's sex. Touch his pubic mound and give your blessing, saying "May the door to your pleasure open wide for you this day."

Then anoint Shiva's heart center with oil, saying "May our hearts merge in love and trust."

Touch his third eye lightly with your middle finger, saying "May your orgasm expand your vision and understanding."

Yang can function only with the cooperation of yin, and yin can grow only in the presence of yang.

—*The Yellow Emperor*

Shakti, when the blessing is complete, help Shiva to lie comfortably amid the cushions in a half-sitting position. Sit between Shiva's legs. Slide your legs under his and put pillows on your thighs so he can rest his knees on them (see illustration). Or you may prefer to kneel, Japanese style, with a cushion under your thighs. Some women like to sit at the man's side, close to his body. Some prefer to use a massage table so that the man is lying down while the woman is standing.

In my experience, however, the most intimate position is when Shiva reclines on big pillows and Shakti sits between his legs, close to the Vajra, although you may need to change the position of your legs from time to time during the exercise.

Shakti, slowly open Shiva's robe, exposing the front of his body.

Begin to caress his whole body, touching him everywhere, encouraging him to breathe deeply with his mouth open. Breathe in synchronicity with him.

If Shiva seems too serious, give him a tickle session, blow in his ear, nibble an ear lobe, lightly bite his throat, suck his toe, tease his body with your breasts, run your hair over him, creating an atmosphere of lightness and humor, inspiring him to trust and relax.

Massage his chest, gently squeezing and teasing his nipples. Then slide your hands under the small of his back and vigorously massage the sacrum area. Many sexual tensions are held in the V-shaped point where the back meets the buttocks.

Cup Shiva's testicles, his balls, in one hand, touching his perineum with the tip of the middle finger. In this position, the flat of your hand can press against the Vajra (see illustration). Place your other hand on Shiva's heart center, in the middle of his chest.

In this position, gaze softly into his eyes, bringing all your love and attention to this being. He is the only one, the special one, and all your energy is focused on him. Allow this moment to wash away any intruding thoughts of distractions.

Shiva, open yourself to the love of your partner. Feel yourself becoming receptive, like a glass waiting to be filled with rich, dark wine.

STAGE 2: STROKES FOR STIMULATING THE VAJRA
Shakti, when you feel ready, ask Shiva, "Shall we start the session now?" If Shiva says "yes," you can begin to stimulate his Vajra, using all or any of the following strokes.

The Twelve O'Clock Stroke   This stroke directly caresses the Vajra.

Caress upward, from the balls to the tip of the Vajra, with the flat part of your hands and fingers, giving alternating strokes with your left and right hand in a smooth, continuous series of movements. Shiva's Vajra should be lying on his belly for this stroke. Use lots of oil.

This stroke is particularly pleasurable because Shakti's hands are passing over the frenulum, on the underside of Shiva's Vajra, where the head meets the shaft.

Growing the Stalk   Cover Shiva's Vajra with lots of oil. Hold the base of the Vajra with one hand, pressing

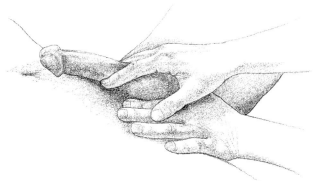

Twelve-o'clock stroke

Strokes for stimulating the Vajra

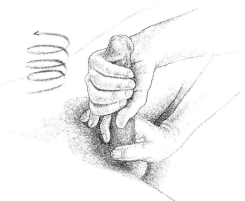

Spiraling the stalk

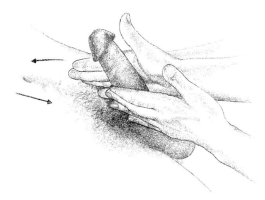

Making fire

down slightly, then stroke straight upward from the base to the tip with the other hand.

Spiraling the Stalk   Hold the Vajra at the base with one hand, then turn your other hand around the Vajra in a circular movement, beginning at the bottom and winding your way up to the head. When you get to the top, caress the whole head with the palm of your hand, using plenty of oil.

The Carousel   Hold the Vajra with both hands and rotate them in opposite directions around the stalk. Move your torso backward and forward in harmony with the movement of the hands.

Shakti, this stroke involves your whole body. Rock backward and forward from your pelvis, inhaling and ex-haling deeply as you move back and forth, while rotating your hands around the Vajra.

Doing this stroke while looking in the eyes of your partner can be both delightful and playful, and has been likened to riding a carousel in an amusement park.

Making Fire   With the palms of your hands held vertically, facing each other on either side of the Vajra, press against the stalk and rub your hands backward and forward as if trying to start a fire by rubbing a stick. Start at the base of the Vajra, work up to the head and then down again.

Drumming the Vajra　Hold the head of Shiva's Vajra against his belly with the index and middle fingers of one hand, then lightly dance the fingers of your other hand over the back surface of the Vajra. You can play it like a small drum, using the whole underside of your fingers, not just the fingertips.

Stroking without the Hood　If Shiva has not been circumcised the head will be protected by his foreskin. It's nice to stimulate the head with the foreskin covering it. When he gets more excited, gently pull back the foreskin and directly stimulate the head, lightly massaging up and down with lots of lubricant.

STAGE 3: BUILDING SEXUAL AROUSAL

Now it is time for Shiva to begin a steady climb toward his first sexual peak. The easiest way to do this is through prolonged, rhythmic stimulation of the Vajra.

Shakti, liberally oil Shiva's Vajra and then hold the base with one hand. With your other hand grasp the stalk, surrounding it with your palm and fingers, and begin to stroke the stalk firmly up and down. This is the basic stroke that most men need to rise toward their sexual climax, but there are several variations.

Your stroke can move up and down the stalk, or it can include the head as well. You can alternate between stroking the stalk and stroking the stalk and head together.

Another option is to find a stroke that allows your thumb to press on the frenulum as your hand moves from the stalk to the head. At the end of the upward movement there is a kind of "snapping" or "flicking" movement with the wrist that can send a delightful pulse of pleasure into the frenulum.

Shiva, teach Shakti the strokes that really do it for you. Give her as much feedback as possible on the rhythm, intensity, and speed that give you most pleasure, so that she can create exactly the right strokes.

Shakti, some men like to have a steady, ongoing stroke that is strong and quick, while others like more variation. Don't get discouraged if Shiva doesn't peak right away, or if he doesn't get excited quickly. Now he is in the receptive mode and it may be more difficult for him to peak. Stay centered, have trust in yourself, becoming familiar with the process of stimulating your man for long periods of time. Settle into a rhythm of stimulating Shiva's Vajra.

Many women are not used to giving strong, rapid stimulation in this way, so listen to Shiva's guidance. Let him tell you what pressure, speed, and intensity he likes. If he is not speaking, ask him, "Is this okay?" "Is this exciting?" You need close and accurate communication.

Shiva, you may come to a place during stimulation when your penis is getting insensitive. If you're not feeling much, ask Shakti to leave your Vajra alone and massage your body from your Vajra toward your chest, spreading the energy toward your heart center. Then, after a few minutes, she can gradually come back to the Vajra, teasing the stalk, tickling the frenulum, caressing the head, before resuming rhythmic stimulation.

STAGE 4: PEAKING WITHOUT EJACULATING

Shakti, you are now moving from a general pleasuring of Shiva's Vajra to a precise method of stimulation that brings him close to ejaculation, without crossing the point of no return.

Build up the pace, stimulating his Vajra in a more dynamic way that brings him toward his orgasmic peak.

Shiva, now is the time to become really sexy and aroused, reaching toward your preejaculation peak. Focus all your attention on the sensations in your Vajra. Go for your lust, your excitement. Move your body. Thrust upward with your pelvis so you can feel Shakti's strokes on your Vajra even more acutely. Exhale strongly through your mouth, pushing your energy down into your genitals. If it is helpful, do the PC Pump, squeezing the muscles around your perineum and anus in short, strong, rhythmic spasms.

Shakti, bring Shiva to an "almost climax," not quite reaching his point of ejaculation. This means that you need to cease all stimulation for at least three to five seconds before the ejaculatory reflex sets in. The following signs help you know when Shiva is getting close to orgasm:

1. His thigh and stomach muscles begin to tense.

2. His back arches, pushing his pelvis closer to you.

3. The testicles contract upward toward the body.

4. His breathing pattern changes. Some men breathe noticeably faster, others slower.

5. The head of the Vajra becomes darker in color.

6. The Vajra becomes very hard, the veins bulge, as it becomes engorged with blood.

7. The Vajra tends to feel incredibly alive and energized.

8. There is frequent emission of a clear fluid from the opening of the urethra.

Shiva, when you feel that your level of sexual excitement is peaking and bringing you very close to ejaculation, use the code word you have arranged with Shakti. Say "Stop!"

Shakti, stop all stimulation of the Vajra. Press strongly into Shiva's perineum point with the index and middle finger of one hand, while holding the Vajra with the other. This will help him not to ejaculate.

Or, if necessary, you can press firmly with the thumbs and fingers of both hands on the Vajra stalk, just below the head. This technique is normally used only when Shiva has come too close to ejaculation and needs extra help in preventing it.

Shiva, breathe strongly and deeply, filling your lungs with air, helping the energy spread through your pelvis. Allow your whole body to relax each time you exhale, letting go of control, becoming receptive to the exquisite sensations in your genitals.

Shakti, your partner's desire to ejaculate will pass in a few moments. When you feel he is ready, ask "Shall I begin again?"

If Shiva says "yes," begin to stimulate his Vajra once

more. Over the next twenty to thirty minutes, bring him to a peak of sexual pleasure between three and six times.

If you both feel it is appropriate, you can end the session by giving Shiva's Vajra the final blessing and stimulating him all the way to the point of ejaculation.

Shiva and Shakti, sit or lie quietly together for a few minutes, absorbing the powerful experience you have shared.

Shiva, be sure to express your appreciation to Shakti for giving you so much pleasure. Reward her with a Melting Hug.

Share your experiences of what happened during the practice.

Close with a Heart Salutation.

Five Basic Points for Vajra Stimulation

Here are five basic points to remember when stimulating the Vajra:

1. Develop a good heart connection.

2. Start with playful, erotic foreplay: including stroking whole body.

3. Explore various strokes on the Vajra.

4. Practice rhythmic stimulation.

5. Come to several peaks without ejaculating.

Pointers

DROPPING THE "STRONG, SILENT" IMAGE

Shiva, as you probably know, men are not used to talking before, during, or after sex, so it is quite a challenge for you to move away from this "strong, silent" mode of male behavior toward an easy attitude of continuous communication.

One good tip is to keep your eyes open, to look at your partner while she pleasures you. Or, if you feel you must close your eyes at certain times in order fully to enjoy the sensations arising in your sexual organ, alternate between keeping them closed and looking at your Shakti.

It is very important that you be willing to describe what you are feeling, otherwise Shakti will not be able to develop the skills she needs to bring you to higher and higher ecstatic peaks. Talk to her about each different stroke: how it feels, how you want to be touched, whether the pressure should be strong or light, what kind of stimulation turns you on most.

Resist the temptation to say "That's fine" to everything Shakti does, as this does not help to build her skills. But remember to stay positive in your communication, respecting Shakti's willingness to give to you.

Shakti, when your man begins to relax and enjoy himself, sinking into a blissful trance, you may feel that

Sexual erection is comparable to water and fire. Water and fire can kill a man or a woman, or help them, depending upon how they are used.

—PAO
The Plane Master

101

you don't want to disturb him by asking questions. But it is important to keep communicating, Ask short, simple questions that can be answered with a few words, like "Does this feel good?" "Do you want it stronger?" "Shall I try something different?"

A Successful First Experience

A good experience of expanded orgasmic states comes from a subtle interplay of technique, creativity, and communication. Bob and Sarah, a couple who had been together for seven years, had experimented with several Tantric techniques but had never done the exercise I have just described. Bob tells the story of their first experience:

> I had a shower while Sarah prepared the space. Earlier, I told her about Margo's idea to use olive oil as a lubricant and we both agreed to try it. But, just in case, we had a variety of oil-based and water-based lubricants handy.
>
> I put on my favorite bathrobe and Sarah led me to the bedroom. She had covered the bed with a white satin sheet and placed a towel on the spot where I would sit, in case any oil dripped on the bed. An array of large cushions was stacked against the end of the bed so that I could recline in a half-sitting, half-lying position, in a very kingly manner. Music was playing and the atmosphere was relaxing and welcoming.

It felt very good to lie there, watching Sarah take off her robe to reveal her shapely body. She did a spontaneous dance for me, which was just delightful, then came and sat between my legs. We did a Heart Salutation and placed our hands on each other's hearts. Then she anointed the three chakras with oil, making an invocation at each one, and started to massage my whole body lightly.

Although I enjoyed this, I could also feel that I was getting impatient, thinking "Okay, this is nice, but when do we get to the real thing? When is she going to touch my Vajra?"

Sensing this, Sarah asked me "Bob, are you worried about the time?" And I had to admit it was true, because because we'd agreed on an hour for the session and quite a lot of time had gone by already, so I was anxious that the really pleasurable part of the session would be cut short.

Once it was clear what was bothering me we easily solved the problem by agreeing to continue the session until we had completed all the stages of the exercise, which we figured would take between ninety to one hundred twenty minutes. Then I could really relax and enjoy each moment.

This was also important for Sarah. She told me that she really needed to feel a heart connection between us in order to enjoy what she was doing, and my impatience was making this connection difficult.

I liked it when she cupped my genitals in her hand and tuned in, gazing into my eyes. Then she began to stroke and pretty soon my Vajra was erect.

I soon realized that I liked a lot of oil on my Vajra. The more oil, the more erotic and pleasurable the sensations, so I often said "more oil" and Sarah would oblige.

Then she moved into an exploration of the different strokes. It was just delightful for me to have all this attention focused on my penis. For once, I didn't have to worry about giving pleasure to Sarah. I could just bathe in the luxury of her total attention and the sensations in my Vajra.

For Sarah, it was important to have the freedom to adapt each stroke to her own style, and some worked better than others. A favorite of ours was the carousel, which was not only erotic but also playful because the rocking and twisting motion really did remind us of riding a carousel at a fairground.

Throughout this time I felt very sexual, my Vajra was hard, but I didn't have any trouble preventing ejaculation. I wasn't close to orgasm, and this was probably due to the fact that once Sarah began to caress my Vajra I became very relaxed, enjoying the whole show.

But this became a problem when it was time for me

to move toward an orgasmic peak. Sarah used the basic stroke, but I didn't feel any great excitement. I offered to show her how to do it, but then I found that it didn't make much difference. I was hard, but not able to approach the peak.

At this point, Sarah said that she didn't really enjoy doing the repetitive basic stroke for very long, so she started playing around with a whole variety of strokes, using lots of oil.

In response, my body started to move around in a very sensual kind of way. At first, I held back, embarrassed, thinking "well, this is how women behave when they're turned on, not guys," but it felt so good that I just gave in to it.

Sarah was doing all kinds of strokes on my Vajra and I was pushing my hips up toward her, arching my back, running my hands over my face and chest, sighing, moaning, grunting and suddenly I was getting really turned on, really excited.

To my surprise, Sarah was also getting turned on. She told me later that my movements released a surge of male energy through my genitals that she found very arousing. So she was very happy, pouring oil over my Vajra and my body, letting me press my hips against her stomach while she rubbed my Vajra between her breasts and squeezed my nipples.

It was getting pretty wild and exciting for both of us. I came to my first peak and said "now" and we both stopped moving. There was an exquisite sensation in my Vajra, but I could also feel how my physical movements had opened up energy channels inside my body. My pelvis, belly, chest, and throat all felt more open, more alive, so the pleasure wasn't just local. It was spreading.

I came to a peak about four to five times without ejaculating and then told Sarah that I wanted to go for the full orgasm. She was so excited by this time that she was squirming her buttocks on the sheet while pleasuring my Vajra, so with one hand I dipped my fingers in the oil and reached between her legs, pleasuring her clitoris while she brought me to a final climax.

We both came at the same time, laughing wildly, rocked by spasms of pleasure, with semen and oil running all over us. It was great. I have rarely enjoyed myself so much, and afterward we felt very loving and affectionate toward each other, like having a new honeymoon.

Heading into a Forbidden Sexual Zone

Now that the "front" part of Shiva's sexual organs has been well taken care of, it's time to discover ways of generating sexual excitement in the "back" part. In the following exercise, Shakti will be massaging the perineum area between Shiva's testicles and anus, thereby stimulating the prostate gland that lies just beneath the surface (see illustration of male anatomy).

Before introducing the practice, it will be helpful to examine some of the social attitudes that inhibit a man's ability to experience pleasure in the prostate and anal areas. You will find that you are working against a lifetime of taboos and opposing ideas and impulses.

From early on, often in a premature manner, children are taught a form of "toilet training" that includes contracting the anal sphincter muscle and the muscles around the prostate in order to hold back their stool. Should they fail in this endeavor, an attitude of disgust and condemnation is almost invariably directed toward them, conveying a strong message that this kind of behavior is unacceptable. Soon, they learn that this area of the body is somehow dirty.

In addition, it has been established that emotional denial, especially denial of anger, is closely associated with the contraction of anal muscles. For example, your boss has been nasty or rude to you at work, and you find yourself feeling very angry but unable to express it. Automatically, you tighten the muscles around your anus. As you do so, your breathing tends to become shallow, your stomach gets tense, and all energy flow to the anal and pelvic area is cut off.

A third source of tension derives from the universally accepted "missionary position" style of lovemaking in which the man, lying on top of the woman, makes repeated thrusts, using his pelvis to propel his Vajra into the Yoni in a dynamic and powerful way. This kind of lovemaking can be great fun and highly pleasurable, but when used habitually, in a strong, repetitive way, it creates layers of tension around the buttocks and anus, especially in the area of the prostate where the thrusting impulse originates.

Fear of homosexuality provides yet another source of tension. The idea that pleasure can be gained from caressing and stimulating this area may feel threatening to a man who has cultivated an image of being strongly heterosexual.

Unpleasant and insensitive prostate examinations, which nearly all men have to endure at some time, also create tension. The impact of a doctor's finger being suddenly rammed into your anus lasts well beyond the initial shock and hurt. Moreover, in recent years, the prostate gland has become a major source of medical concern with the rising incidence of prostate cancer.

For all these reasons, the anal area has become difficult terrain to explore and enjoy. But this traumatic social conditioning can be changed. There is a new challenge ahead: to relax this tense, forbidden area and allow it to be healed, to be nourished, to become a source of great pleasure independently of any cultural judgments or taboos. It is time for all of us to recognize that this part of the male body needs as much care and attention as any other part.

EXERCISE: STIMULATING THE PROSTATE EXTERNALLY

Purpose and benefits

To deepen the male partner's experience of the receptive aspect of his sexuality by stimulating his prostate gland. The prostate is stimulated externally by massaging the perineum area, between the testicles and the anus. This practice paves the way for an experience of multiple, implosive orgasms as opposed to the explosive orgasm of normal ejaculation.

Stimulation of the prostate gives you, Shiva, an experience comparable to the female G-Spot orgasm. You will experience how sexual pleasure can spread from your Vajra to your prostate in the same way that a woman's pleasure spreads from her clitoris to her G-Spot.

Combined stimulation of your Vajra and prostate allows you to connect two distinct types of pleasure: outer-directed sexual sensations and inner-directed ones.

When you ejaculate, the muscles around your prostate have a reflex response, a series of pulsations or contractions that help to eject semen out through the urethra. By stimulating the prostate, you can experience a subtle, ongoing stream of pleasurable sensations that requires no ejaculation.

Preparations

- Be gentle and loving when exploring this area. When you receive a prostate massage there may be mild sensations of temporary discomfort, which are natural when sensitizing a neglected area of the body. It is best not to work directly on the prostate for more than five to seven minutes in the first few sessions.

- If you have recently experienced inflammation of the prostate, or had an infection in this area, or have a medical history of prostate problems, you should not do this massage unless you receive permission from your doctor.

- Shiva, be sure that you take a shower and thoroughly clean your genitals and anus. One of the most important aids to easy and comfortable prostate stimulation is for both partners to know that the anus is clean.

- ✹ Shakti, you may want to adopt the attitude of a medical student, focusing on achieving skillful stimulation through experimenting and sharing information.

- ✹ Shakti, create the Sacred Space while Shiva readies himself to receive the massage.

- ✹ Make sure your fingernails are short and smooth.

- ✹ If you wish, you can wear latex gloves as an added hygienic precaution.

- ✹ Use a lot of oil-based lubricant.

- ✹ Allow forty-five minutes for this exercise.

STAGE 1: FOREPLAY WITH VIGOROUS MASSAGE

Shakti, welcome Shiva to your Sacred Space.

Begin with a Heart Salutation and a long Melting Hug.

Shakti, take off your beloved's robe and help him lie down on his stomach. If you wish, you can work on a massage table.

Begin to give Shiva a deep, dynamic massage all round his buttocks, including his lower back, sacrum, and the tops of his thighs. This is an important preparation for approaching the prostate. Make your massaging movements from your hara—your center of balance, below the navel—using your whole body.

Be playful. Enjoy yourself. Massaging the buttocks can be rather like kneading dough in a bakery.

End by placing one hand on each buttock and shaking them vigorously for two to three minutes, then stroke down the backs of Shiva's legs from his buttocks to his feet. Tap the soles of his feet, grounding the energy.

Experience your individuality as a healthy leaf. You feel the sap flowing from the vine of your innermost self.

—The Bird Tribe Book

STAGE 2: ROUSING THE THUNDERBOLT (VAJRA STIMULATION)

Shakti, when you have finished, as Shiva to turn onto his back and recline in the half-lying position, propped against cushions or pillows.

Take time to tune in to Shiva, cupping his sexual organ with one hand while placing your other hand on his heart center. Gaze lovingly into his eyes, feeling the trust and excitement flowing between you. Tell him something wonderful, like "This is all for you. I love you; just allow yourself to receive."

Breathe deeply and harmoniously together.

Shatki, as with the stimulation of your G-Spot, it is important for Shiva to be thoroughly aroused sexually before you begin to caress his prostate. The engorgement of the Vajra helps any tensions around the prostate area to soften and relax.

Lubricate Shiva's Vajra with plenty of oil and begin to stimulate this power scepter in the ways you have already learned. Go through your repertoire of skills and strokes, bringing orgasmic delight to your partner, then settle into a steady rhythm that brings Shiva to a peak of sexual excitement.

Shiva, use your code word to stop just before the point of no return.

Shakti, cease stimulation, letting your hand rest on his Vajra.

Shiva, relax, breath slowly and deeply, allowing your orgasmic sensations to be absorbed and spread through your pelvis. Now you are ready to move to the prostate.

STAGE 3: MASSAGING THE PERINEUM AREA

Shakti, after stimulating your partner's Vajra for fifteen to twenty minutes, bringing him to several peaks, ask him, "Now I would like to focus on your prostate. Is this okay with you?"

If he says "yes," begin to explore the perineum area.

Shakti, begin by stroking the skin surface between Shiva's testicles and anus. Feel the mound just beneath the testicles that forms the root of Shiva's Vajra, then trace it back toward the anus, noticing when your fingers start to push into a soft, fleshy area. This is the perineum, where the prostate is located inside the body.

Feel the two big sitting bones of Shiva's pelvis, at the bottom of his buttocks, and trace these down toward the perineum. Again, you will find yourself pushing into a soft, fleshy area.

Shiva, you may discover that, because this area is not often touched, it may be quite insensitive. Give Shakti plenty of time to find her way around. The more familiar she is with this territory, the more pleasure she can give you later on.

Shakti, the following strokes are designed to loosen and relax the perineal area, bringing sensitivity and aliveness, releasing tension. You may wish to place a small cushion under Shiva's buttocks to make the area more accessible.

Pressing with Fingers Shakti, press with your fingers in the area between the testicles and the anus, feeling where it is hard, where it is soft. You may find that you can press quite deeply and strongly in the soft area that covers the prostate.

Use pressure from your index and middle finger to

find the most pleasurable point, experimenting while your partner guides you: "Yes here, now try further up, down a bit . . ."

Shiva, as Shakti starts to massage, begin the PC Pump, rhythmically contracting the muscles around your perineum and anus as you inhale deeply through your mouth. Keep your throat open.

As you inhale, imagine that you are breathing down into your heart. As you exhale, imagine that you are pushing the energy down toward your pelvis. This will help to relax tension in every part of your body.

Guide Shakti. Tell her how it feels, how much pressure you need.

Pressing with Knuckles Shakti, make a fist and begin to press gently with your knuckles into the whole perineal area. Maintain close communication with Shiva, asking him "Is this strong enough? How about if I do it like this?"

Once you know the point and the pressure, you will remember later on how to use a finger or knuckle to prevent Shiva from ejaculating in states of high arousal.

Vibrating with Fist Make a fist and press with the flat area—between the first and second set of knuckles—against the perineal floor. Shake your fist, vibrating the

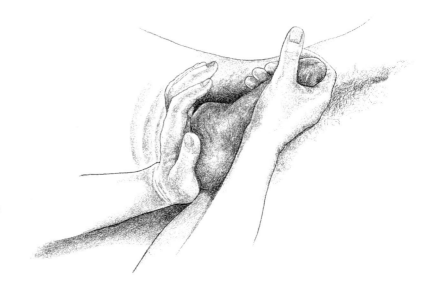

External stimulation of the
prostate gland: vibrations
applied on the perineum
while pleasing the penis

External stimulation of the
prostate: vibrating and
pressing the fist on the
perineum

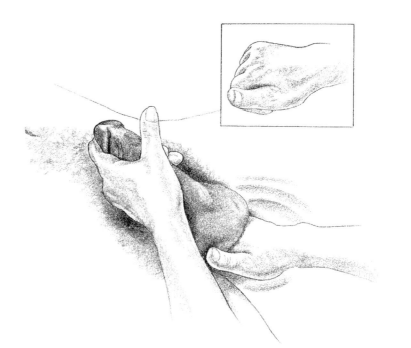

whole area, sending tremors pulsing into the perineum. With your free hand, massage Shiva's chest and belly.

Encourage Shiva to move his body, push forward with his pelvis, let out sounds, so that the vibration can expand and spread into his pelvis and chest.

Vibrating with Both Hands Slide your fingers under the base of Shiva's spine (the coccyx area) so that the heel of your hand presses against his perineum. Rest your left hand on Shiva's lower belly. Now you are holding his entire lower pelvis between your two hands. Using your whole body, moving from your hara, shake your hands so that this area vibrates.

STAGE 4: BUILDING SEXUAL AROUSAL

Shakti, now that you have energized the area around Shiva's perineum you can experiment with stimulating the Vajra and prostate together.

First, oil the Vajra and begin stroking the stalk, using your favorite style, bringing this magic wand to a state of erect alertness.

When the Vajra is erect, stimulate the perineum with your free hand, pressing firmly with your fingers or knuckles. Massage the perineum with a circular motion, or rubbing up and down, or giving quick pulsations on the spot.

Begin to massage Shiva's Vajra and the perineum area at the same pace. This steady, blended rhythm can help him build sexual arousal without getting too focused on the sensations in his Vajra.

The philosopher's stone transforms base metal into gold. In the heart of the jewel, love and passion can transform one into pure awareness.

—*Tantric Alchemy*

Here is a good stroke to try: Take the Vajra in your right hand, holding it at the base. With your left hand, make a circle with your thumb and index finger containing the scrotal sack, just under the Vajra so that the whole sack lies in the palm of your hand as you press against the perineum with the flat part of your fingers, between the first and second set of knuckles.

Experiment with this position, stroking the Vajra with your right hand while vibrating the perineum with your left.

Shiva, tell Shakti how it feels—what degree of intensity, pressure, and speed you need.

Here is an excellent tip: Shiva, in the initial stages, while Shakti is familiarizing herself with external prostate massage, you may want to stimulate your Vajra yourself. You can bring yourself to a sexual peak, expanding your awareness to include the new sensations created by Shakti. This can be very exciting for you and also gives Shakti more freedom to focus on the perineum area.

Shakti, if you find it difficult to caress the perineum while directly facing it, ask Shiva to part his legs wider so that you can sit at right angles to his genital area.

STAGE 5: COMBINED PEAKING

Shakti, bring Shiva to an orgasmic peak with strong, combined stimulation of the Vajra and perineum.

Shiva, really go for your pleasure, breathing strongly, rubbing your perineum against Shakti's hands by pushing down with your pelvis, moving your body, making sounds. Focus on your sexual sensations and seek to heighten them, encouraging Shakti to stimulate you in whatever way brings added excitement.

At the peak, stop, use the code word, cease all stimulation.

Shiva, relax your body, breathe slowly and deeply, focusing on the delightful sensations that are pulsing through your pelvis. Allow these sensations, even if they seem strange and new to you. Give in to them. Feel how the Vajra and prostate are complementing each other in this orgasmic dance.

Repeat this process as many times as you wish.

Bring the session to a close with a Melting Hug.

Shiva, thank Shakti for her willingness to give you new dimensions of pleasure.

Take a short break and then give feedback.

Five Basic Points for Massaging the Perineum
Here are five basic points to remember when stimulating
the prostate externally:

1. Begin with vigorous massage around the buttocks.

2. Stimulate the Vajra before approaching the perineum
   area.

3. Explore various strokes on the perineum.

4. Give rhythmic, combined stimulation to the Vajra
   and perineum.

5. Practice peaking without ejaculating.

Pointers
BLENDING INTENSE EXCITEMENT WITH RECEPTIVITY
Shiva, the first problem you may encounter when Shakti
massages your perineum area is that the more relaxed you
become around your anus and prostate the less excitement
you may feel in your Vajra.

You can counter this tendency by asking Shakti to
continue to stimulate your Vajra while massaging your
perineum, but if you do lose your erection there is no

need to worry: this is a stage to pass through on the way to greatly enhanced orgasmic pleasure.

The focus of your attention should not be on maintaining an erection, but on exploring and enjoying the new sensations that are being created around your prostate area. Here, Shakti is helping you to open the receptive aspect of your sexuality.

When, with Shakti's help, you have acquired the knack of blending intense sexual excitement with relaxation and receptivity, you will be able to experience ongoing orgasmic pleasure that can last up to ten to twenty minutes. This happens when the area around your prostate and anus is relaxed and sensitized.

Special Hygienic Procedure

We are about to move into the third and final phase of exploring the alchemy of male orgasm, in which Shakti will stimulate Shiva's prostate internally, by gently penetrating into the anal canal with her fingers and massaging the gland directly.

Before doing so, however, there is a special hygienic procedure that I encourage Shiva to practice. Many women are accustomed to using a vaginal douche, but there is a certain taboo about using the same technique for the anal passage, especially among heterosexual men. Such practices may stir uneasy feelings about homosexuality, or the risk of being thought a "sissy" by your partner.

However, I can assure you that this simple and straightforward method of cleaning your rectum will be greatly appreciated by your partner. She will be grateful for your hygienic care, for the knowledge that her role in this exercise is being fully supported by you. Moreover, a cleansing douche, or enema, using lukewarm water, will sensitize the area around your prostate and help you feel more pleasure.

Remember, no matter how shocking or embarrassing it may seem, this gesture of cleaning your rectal passage is really no different from cleaning the basement of your house. You are cleansing and purifying yourself of "emotional garbage"—in the form of tensions and armoring created by withheld anger, early toilet training, etc.—that has been stored in this area of the body since childhood.

In my experience of introducing many couples to this practice I have found that, in addition to enhancing male sexual pleasure, internal massage can help to soothe and reduce hemorrhoids; it also keeps the prostate gland healthy and energized.

EXERCISE: STIMULATING
THE PROSTATE INTERNALLY

Purpose and benefits

To provide Shiva with the ultimate, blended orgasmic sensations by internally stimulating his prostate while at the same time stimulating his Vajra. This exercise gives Shiva the Tantric experience of balancing his own male and female energies: strong male energy is being aroused in his Vajra while more receptive, feminine sensations are being generated in his prostate area.

After this experience, Shiva can understand Shakti more fully, for now he knows what it is like to be pleasured through penetration.

Another benefit of this practice is enhanced sensitivity in Shiva's Vajra during contact with Shakti's Yoni in lovemaking.

It also provides the deepest and most powerful sensations of male orgasm that will prove invaluable in the practice of sexual magic.

Shiva, in this exercise you go to the very roots of male creative power, into the area where semen mixes with prostatic fluids, honoring and caring for this part of your earthly temple. In so doing, you will feel the added excitement of discovering an entirely new area of pleasure that has been previously ignored.

Linga and Shakti are shaped to one another, for how else could new life be born? Desire yokes man and woman in one passionate union.

—Kama Sutra

Preparations

- Shakti, for an internal prostate massage it is important that your fingernails be closely trimmed and filed to a smooth roundness, with no hangnails or sharp corners.

- You can purchase latex gloves to cover your fingers, should you wish to use them for the internal stimulation of the prostate. This will also protect the delicate and sensitive internal tissues from any rough spots on your fingers.

- Have tissues or paper towels handy.

- Shiva, to clean your anal canal, purchase a small or "travel" enema bag at any major drugstore. Or ask Shakti to buy it for you. Use two cups of warm water, adding a few drops of a natural dermicide (such as essential oil of lavender) for added cleanliness. When you have finished, take a shower and prepare to be pampered.

- Shakti, it is your job to prepare the Sacred Space. For this delicate exercise, take special care to create a nurturing, protective environment for Shiva.

- Allow ninety minutes for this exercise.

STAGE 1: AROUSING THE VAJRA

Shakti, lead Shiva into the Sacred Space.

Begin with a strong rhythmic dance, jumping up and down, grounding the energy so that you both feel energized and centered.

Shakti, invite Shiva to recline on large pillows and sit close to his sexual organs, as in the previous exercise.

As with the external stimulation of the prostate, it is good to begin by stimulating Shiva's Vajra. This will engorge the area around the prostate with blood, relax any tensions, and increase Shiva's awareness of this invisible gland.

Make sure Shiva becomes thoroughly aroused, bringing him to a peak of sexual excitement by stroking his Vajra. Come close to the point of no return at least once.

It is important that you maintain contact with the Vajra throughout your exploration of the prostate, giving occasional stimulation, as this will help Shiva feel secure in his male sexuality and trust what you are doing.

STAGE 2: KNOCKING ON THE DOOR

Shakti, oil the anus and the cleft between Shiva's buttocks. Begin to slowly massage and caress the external part of the anus. Use plenty of lubricant. This can be a new and exciting sensation for Shiva but it can also be very scary, so don't be in a hurry.

Ask Shiva how it feels.

Shiva, if you are feeling nervous, do the PC Pump and rock your pelvis back and forth, breathing strongly through your mouth, making sounds. This dynamic preparation will help blood flow to the area, bringing fresh energy and vitality, and help dissolve any tensions.

Shakti, when you feel ready, leave your fingers on Shiva's anus, waiting at the door, and ask "Is it okay to move in?"

If Shiva says "yes," press gently on the anal opening with your index finger, using a lot of lubrication.

Shiva, by gently doing the PC Pump, squeezing the muscles around your anus and perineum, you will find that this movement sucks Shakti's index finger inside the anal opening.

STAGE 3: PENETRATING THE ANUS

Shakti, very slowly penetrate into the anus with your middle or index finger. As you do so, you may feel Shiva's sphincter muscle (the muscle surrounding the anal opening) become tense and rigid. If this happens, pause and wait for the area to relax. As the tension passes, wiggle your finger very gently for a few moments, then penetrate a little deeper. Go very slowly and sensitively, allowing the area to relax.

When your finger has penetrated about one inch inside, bend it in a crooked position and begin to rim the anal sphincter from within, pressing all around the anal opening from the inside. Press slowly. After a while, you can also begin to vibrate your finger a little.

Shiva, breathe deeply through your mouth while Shakti massages the inner rim of your sphincter muscle. If you find many tensions in this area, you may feel you need to spend one or more sessions just relaxing this area. Do not try to push past any discomfort or pain. Be very gentle with yourself. Guide Shakti so that penetration and stimulation happen at a pace and rhythm that is comfortable to you.

STAGE 4: ENCOUNTERING THE PROSTATE

Shakti, you will know that it is okay to penetrate more deeply when you feel Shiva's anus is relaxed and comfortable. Now the muscles are getting used to your touch. Your penetration is welcome.

Keep exploring inside the anus. Ask Shiva "How does this feel?" Stay in close communication with each other.

Move your finger deeper into the anal passage, curving it slightly upward, until you encounter a round, firm body of issue that is shaped like a chestnut. This is the prostate.

Shiva, you will probably notice a deep, unfamiliar sensation—it can be pleasurable, or it may just feel strange—when Shakti's finger presses against your prostate. When this happens, let her know that she has found the right spot.

Take plenty of time to explore the entire area.

Again, I would like to assure Shiva that there is no need to worry if you lose your erection. It is more important to develop a mutual understanding of the territory.

Help Shakti locate the prostate and become familiar with its shape, size, and the degree to which she can press on it. Remember, you are the guide.

Stage 5: Stimulating the Prostate

Shiva, in the beginning, the sensations you feel when Shakti presses on your prostate may not necessarily be pleasurable. They may feel strange. Or you may not feel much at all. Like the G-Spot, stimulation of the prostate sometimes takes two or three sessions to become a pleasurable experience.

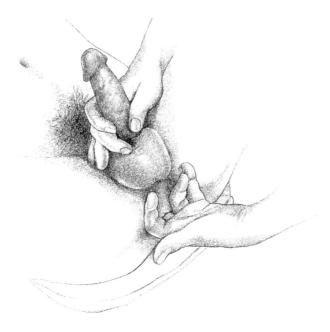

Simultaneous stimulation of
the prostate and the penis

Shakti, gently begin to stimulate the whole area of
the prostate. There are three basic strokes for this type of
massage:

1. Make a zigzag motion across the prostate and the surrounding tissue with your finger.

2. Move up and down the prostate with your finger.

3. Keep your finger on the prostate and then lightly
   shake your hand with a trembling motion, vibrating
   the prostate.

Shiva, you may want to do the PC Pump and rotate your pelvis slightly as Shakti stimulates your prostate. Or you may wish to be motionless in order to feel the sensations more accurately.

A good way to release tension is to ask Shakti to vibrate her finger on the prostate, while her other hand stimulates your penis. Or you may wish to focus exclusively on the sensations in your prostate, without stimulating the penis.

Breathe strongly through your mouth, sending fresh energy down to your pelvis. Give Shakti clear communication about how you want her to touch your prostate in order to bring pleasure and sensitivity to this area. Encourage Shakti to use strokes that help you feel your prostate the most.

Shakti, be gentle and use plenty of lubricant. In the beginning, prostate massage should continue no longer than five minutes, and always be aware to stop the practice if there are any painful sensations or a sense of soreness.

STAGE 6: BLENDED STIMULATION OF VAJRA AND PROSTATE
Shiva, when you begin to feel your prostate and become familiar with the territory, you can ask Shakti to begin to expand the experience by simultaneously massaging your prostate and stimulating your Vajra.

How to stimulate the
prostate through the anus

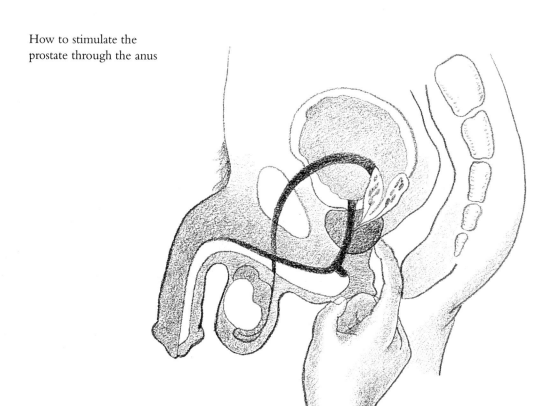

Shakti, experiment with keeping one finger on
Shiva's prostate while, with your other hand, you begin to
stimulate his Vajra. Use plenty of lubricant on both organs.

Here is a combined stroke that I call "Two Friends
Meeting."

Two Friends Meeting   For the purpose of describing this combined stroke, let us imagine that Shakti's right hand is holding the Vajra, while the index finger of her left hand is inside the anus, pressing gently against Shiva's prostate.

Shakti, first, strongly stimulate the Vajra with your right hand, keeping your left index finger motionless on the prostate. When pleasurable sensations begin to spread through the Vajra—it need not be fully erect—start your blended strokes: push inward into the anal passage with your left index finger, passing over and caressing the prostate gland, while at the same time stroking down the stalk of the Vajra with your right hand.

In this way, it seems as if your left index finger inside Shiva's anal canal is going to join your right hand at the base of his Vajra, like two friends meeting. Then, pull back with your finger while stroking up the stalk of the Vajra, like two friends parting, then push inward again while stroking down the Vajra, like two friends meeting, and so on.

You can vary this basic stroke in a number of ways, such as stroking the stalk of the Vajra while pulsing the prostate, or doing a zigzag motion around it.

Shiva, it is your job to give Shakti clear indications, telling her what works, how you want it, what pressures and rhythms feel good. Be as detailed as you like.

Remember, it may take several sessions before your

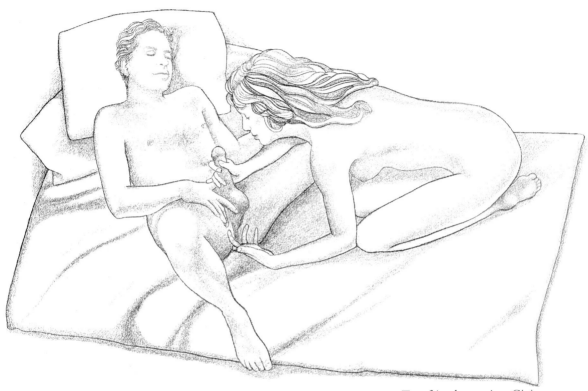

Two friends meeting. Giving the man a blended orgasm by stimulating the penis and the prostate simultaneously

prostate is sensitized and before Shakti has discovered exactly the right strokes to bring you to orgasm, so don't be in a hurry.

A good tip: As with the previous exercise, it can be exciting for Shiva to stimulate his own Vajra while Shakti applies rhythmic stimulation to his prostate. Experiment with this technique.

STAGE 7: MOVING TO A STREAMING ORGASMIC RESPONSE

Shakti, settle into a steady rhythm of simultaneous massage, using a combination of strokes that gives pleasure to Shiva.

Ask Shiva, "Are you ready to peak?"

If he says "yes," increase stimulation in both areas, holding the Vajra firmly, stroking up and down, while vibrating your finger on the prostate.

Shiva, you may want to use the Three Keys to intensify the sexual sensations that are spreading through your genitals and pelvic area: quicken and deepen your breathing, move your body with strong, pelvic thrusts, make sounds that express how you feel. Alternatively, you may want to deeply relax, becoming even more receptive to the exquisite sensations that Shakti is creating.

Go for your ecstasy, go for your pleasure, go for your excitement, in whatever way seems appropriate, reaching toward new orgasmic heights.

When you come to the moment just before ejaculation, use your code word. Say "Now!"

Shakti, cease all stimulation, but keep your finger pressed firmly against Shiva's prostate, as this will help him not to ejaculate.

Shiva, now is the time to totally relax. Feel the orgasmic excitement that has been generated in your whole pelvic area. Give in to these incredible sensations, let them pulsate through your pelvis, your belly, your thighs, spreading out through your body in ripples of orgasmic pleasure. Breathe slowly and deeply.

When you feel ready, began again. Ask Shakti to give blended stimulation to your two pleasure points. Continue in this way, moving toward higher and higher peaks of sexual excitement.

With each peak, the delicious ripples of sexual energy in your pelvic area will become more expanded, more intense, more continuous. Soon, you are likely to experience an ongoing stream of subtle orgasmic excitement that continues inside, with little stimulation required. Allow these orgasmic sensations to take you over. Let them flood your whole body. Become lost in them.

Now there is no need to hold back or control anything, because you are fully surrendered. You are not doing anything. It is just happening, as if you were softly floating, being carried on a river of orgasmic pleasure.

This is the streaming reflex that brings orgasmic ecstasy without any need for ejaculation. It can continue for ten to twenty minutes, even longer.

I never make love in the morning. It's not good for the voice. And besides, you never know who you're going to meet in the afternoon.

—ENRICO CARUSO

Shiva, if you wish to end the session with full orgasmic ejaculation, ask Shakti to give you this final pleasure. Or, if you prefer, lie quietly until your orgasmic streaming sensations fade of their own accord.

Shakti, after a while, ask Shiva if it is okay to retire, then very slowly withdraw your finger from his anus. Take off your latex glove with a paper towel.

After a while, sit up, give each other a Melting Hug.

Shiva, thank Shakti for her generosity in giving you so much pleasure.

Share what you have experienced together.

End with a Heart Salutation.

Five Basic Points for Blended Orgasm

Here are five basic points to remember when stimulating the prostate internally:

1. Stimulate the Vajra.

2. Gently enter the anal canal.

3. Explore strokes on the prostate.

4. Develop blended stimulation of prostate and Vajra.

5. Practice peaking without ejaculating until the orgasmic streaming reflex is triggered.

Pointers

PRACTICE MAKES PERFECT

Shiva and Shakti, while you are learning the techniques of blended stimulation you may come across moments when you feel you are not getting anywhere.

At such times you may think "Oh, it's no good," become discouraged, and feel the whole experiment is fizzling out.

Strong breathing through the mouth is a key. This is what keeps your body energized and helps you stay awake and alert, focusing on each step of the exercise, exploring quiet spaces as well as moments of intense excitement.

You can keep things interesting by experimenting with a variety of strokes. Sometimes it will help to focus exclusively on the Vajra, sometimes on the prostate, sometimes on combined strokes, sometimes on other pleasurable areas such as the entrance to the anal canal.

Supportive and positive communication is very important. Remember to communicate about sensations, strokes, feelings, energy. Avoid criticism, complaints, and impositions.

FEELING HEAT IN THE PROSTATE AREA

Shakti, when you penetrate the anus the first few times
you may get an impression of an intense, fiery heat penetrating your fingers, coming from the prostate or from
some other point inside the anal canal.

Heat is a sign that tension has accumulated at this
point and is now releasing through your touch. If you
keep your finger on the point where the heat is strongest,
vibrating it lightly, you will usually find that the heat disappears after a few minutes and the area is now more relaxed.

POSITION CHANGES

Some men have difficulty lying on their backs for the
whole exercise. They feel overwhelmed and even intimi-
dated by the woman remaining continuously "on top of
them" in a dominant position.

Shakti, if this happens you need to be willing to
change position for a while. For example, Shiva can sit up
while you keep your finger on his prostate. In this way he
can feel that "I am open to you, but now I also want to
show my power, that I am equal to you."

Other men very much enjoy the feeling of being in
the receptive position and are quite happy to remain there
for the whole exercise.

COMBINING ORGASM WITH SEXUAL MAGIC

Shiva and Shakti, you are to be congratulated on breaking through this major cultural taboo, entering through the anus to explore the world of expanded male orgasm, helping Shiva open to ecstatic sensations that most men never knew existed.

Now that both of you have succeeded in expanding your orgasmic potential you are ready to employ this tremendously vital, alive sexual power in the service of your sexual magic.

Resources

SEMINARS / RETREATS

To particiapate in one of Margot Anand's seminars or retreats, please contact

SpiritWorks
Allan Christian
150-24th Street, Suite 407
West Vancouver, BC V7V 4G8
Canada
Phone: 604/922-5622
Fax: 604/922-5623
E-mail: allan_christian@telus.net

Multi Orgasmic Response
For coaching in the Multi Orgasmic Response program, please contact

Kreative World
Kosha Pati and Sohini Genieveve
Phone: 415/789-8339
E-mail: skydancing@kreativeworld. com
Web site: <http://www.skydancingtantra.com>

Margot invites you to visit her Web site, <http://www. skydancing.com>, as well as <http://www.tantra.com>.

ABOUT
THE AUTHOR

MARGOT ANAND is the author of *The Art of Sexual Ecstasy.* She has developed a unique path to sexual bliss called SkyDancing Tantra. She has helped to establish SkyDancing Institutes in eight countries including the USA. She has taught the Love and Ecstasy Trainings around the world to more than ten thousand people for the last fifteen years. Her passion has been to explore and teach that Eros is the source of our creative power and the key to magic: the power to transform, create, and manifest our dream.